Memory and Attention Adaptation Training

Memory and Attention Adaptation Training

A Brief Cognitive Behavioral Therapy for Cancer Survivors

Clinician Manual

Robert J. Ferguson, PhD

Assistant Professor of Medicine, Department of Medicine

Division of Hematology/Oncology

University of Pittsburgh School of Medicine and UPMC Hillman Cancer Center

Pittsburgh, PA, USA

Karen Lee Gillock, PhD

Licensed Clinical Psychologist

Cognitive-Behavioral Therapy

Lebanon, NH, USA

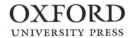

OXFORD

UNIVERSITY PRESS

OXFORD
UNIVERSITY PRESS

Oxford University Press is a department of the University of Oxford. It furthers
the University's objective of excellence in research, scholarship, and education
by publishing worldwide. Oxford is a registered trade mark of Oxford University
Press in the UK and certain other countries.

Published in the United States of America by Oxford University Press
198 Madison Avenue, New York, NY 10016, United States of America.

Library of Congress Cataloging-in-Publication Data
Names: Ferguson, Robert J. (Assistant Professor of medicine), editor. | Gillock, Karen Lee, editor.
Title: Memory and attention adaptation training : a brief cognitive behavioral therapy for cancer survivors
clinician manual / Robert J. Ferguson, Ph.D., Assistant Professor of Medicine,
Division of Hematology/Oncology, University of Pittsburgh School of Medicine and
UPMC Hillman Cancer Center, Karen Lee Gillock, Ph.D., Licensed Clinical
Psychologist, Cognitive-Behavioral Therapy.
Description: New York : Oxford University Press, 2021. |
Includes bibliographical references and index.
Identifiers: LCCN 2020043032 (print) | LCCN 2020043033 (ebook) |
ISBN 978-0-19-752157-1 (paperback) | ISBN 978-0-19-752159-5 (epub) |
ISBN 978-0-19-752160-1
Subjects: LCSH: Cancer—Patients. | Cancer—Patients—Treatment. |
Cognitive therapy. | Memory. | Attention.
Classification: LCC RC265.5 .M46 2021 (print) | LCC RC265.5 (ebook) |
DDC 616.99/4—dc23
LC record available at https://lccn.loc.gov/2020043032
LC ebook record available at https://lccn.loc.gov/2020043033

DOI: 10.1093/med/9780197521571.001.0001

This material is not intended to be, and should not be considered, a substitute for medical or other professional advice.
Treatment for the conditions described in this material is highly dependent on the individual circumstances. And, while
this material is designed to offer accurate information with respect to the subject matter covered and to be current as of
the time it was written, research and knowledge about medical and health issues is constantly evolving and dose schedules
for medications are being revised continually, with new side effects recognized and accounted for regularly. Readers must
therefore always check the product information and clinical procedures with the most up-to-date published product
information and data sheets provided by the manufacturers and the most recent codes of conduct and safety regulation.
The publisher and the authors make no representations or warranties to readers, express or implied, as to the accuracy
or completeness of this material. Without limiting the foregoing, the publisher and the authors make no representations
or warranties as to the accuracy or efficacy of the drug dosages mentioned in the material. The authors and the publisher
do not accept, and expressly disclaim, any responsibility for any liability, loss, or risk that may be claimed or incurred as a
consequence of the use and/or application of any of the contents of this material.

1 3 5 7 9 8 6 4 2

Printed by Integrated Books International, United States of America

Contents

Acknowledgments

MAAT cancer survivor research was funded by grants from the National Cancer Institute (R03 CA90151; R-21CA143619); the Lance Armstrong Foundation; The Beckwith Institute, Pittsburgh, PA; and ongoing research with a grant funded by the National Cancer Institute (R01CA244673). MAAT traumatic brain injury research was funded by the Eunice Kennedy Shriver National Institute of Child Health and Human Development of the National Institutes of Health (R01 HD047242).

We want to express deep gratitude to all research participants and their families for devoting valuable time to MAAT research. Without participants, there can be no research on this treatment program or others in cancer care—thus, no knowledge gained. Thank you.

We also wish to thank all cancer survivors who have undergone MAAT in numerous clinical practices both in the United States and other countries, and who have provided valuable feedback for making improvements in the usability of MAAT.

Use of This Manual

This treatment manual is intended for use by health care professionals trained in cognitive-behavioral therapies (CBTs). Memory and Attention Adaptation Training (MAAT) consists of eight visits and may be considered as a brief CBT or used in a "guided self-help" format. The strategies that the clinician will use are written in great detail to maximize treatment fidelity—or, simply put, consistency in conducting MAAT. Survivors engaged in MAAT use a workbook in conjunction with office or telehealth visits. Clinicians should read the workbook—reproduced in its entirety in Appendix 3—and be familiar with its content.

Each of the eight visits is described in separate sections. *Model dialogue is indicated in italic print. Although clinicians need not quote model dialogue verbatim, critical points that should be made to survivors are presented in this format. This is the convention throughout the manual.* By no means should clinicians read from the manual as they see patients—this has been witnessed by the lead author when training clinicians inexperienced with CBT or using treatment manuals. This is unnatural and belies the warm human interaction that undergirds the positive, collaborative relationship necessary for effective psychological treatment. As an aid to ensure coverage of critical points, there is a checklist for each visit at the beginning of each visit section. These are intended to be photocopied and used during visits. The clinician can keep the checklist on a clipboard during the office or telehealth visit and use the checklist to help guide the agenda. This procedure will also aid treatment fidelity. The same checklists are listed in Appendix 1 along with treatment fidelity rating scales. These "treatment fidelity checklists" can be used by research investigators and independent raters to help evaluate clinicians' adherence to MAAT delivery.

Users of this manual are referred to as "clinicians" because they need not be psychologists. However, it is critical that those licensed health care professionals (such as physicians, nurses, counselors, social workers, or rehabilitation specialists) who want to provide MAAT for cancer survivors or others with mild cognitive dysfunction be well grounded in the principles and applications of CBT. Without this background knowledge, MAAT will be less effective. CBTs such as MAAT involve more than just following a guidebook. While CBT interventions tend to be researched and have a manual to aid delivery of the approach, no manual can substitute for understanding the basics of behavioral analysis, functional contextualism, and social learning theory principles that underlie such interventions.[1] The application of a manual-based treatment in the real world of human behavior requires this knowledge and training experience if patients are to derive full benefit and positive outcomes. Most importantly, fostering a positive, collaborative relationship with the recipient of CBT is key to completing the hard work of behavior change. These points are critical given the ever-increasing pressures of health care cost containment and to ensure the most positive outcomes possible for the expense of treatment.

We suggest strongly that clinicians who are not experienced with CBT seek out adequate supervision and training in CBT approaches before implementing MAAT. There are also informative books about CBT and the behavioral science principles on which it is based[1,2] and the application of CBT in related health care fields.[3,4] With a good grounding in these principles, the clinician will be better equipped to deliver MAAT with optimal effectiveness.

Finally, it is important for the MAAT clinician to be familiar and up to date with the scientific knowledge of cancer-related cognitive impairment (CRCI). The terms "chemobrain" or "chemofog," among others, have been used to describe CRCI, but as explained later, research conducted in the three decades prior to this publication has produced a better understanding of CRCI. A number of triggering factors, such as immune system and inflammatory responses to cancer itself, radiation therapy effects, hormonal changes, stem cell transplantation and other cancer therapies, can affect the cognitive function of survivors. Furthermore, CRCI is just one area among a broad array of survivorship challenges, and it often occurs in the context of family role changes, changes in employment or income, and adjustment to living with the possibility of cancer recurrence. Much of the content to follow in the introduction will discuss the cognitive effects of cancer and its treatments. This discussion is intended as a brief summary and by no means is an exhaustive review of CRCI scientific knowledge. Regardless of the multiple etiological sources of CRCI, MAAT can be used as a CBT to help improve the survivor's daily task function and quality of life. It is hoped that this manual is a thorough yet practical guide for the clinician.

Introduction

Background and Significance of Cancer-Related Cognitive Impairment

The National Cancer Institute's Office of Cancer Survivorship defines a "cancer survivor" as any person diagnosed with cancer in their lifetime from the "time of diagnosis through the balance of his or her life."[5] With advances in early detection and targeted treatments in cancer care, individuals who have been diagnosed with many forms of cancer are living longer than at any other point in history.[6] From 2000 to 2010, U.S. rates of cancer deaths began to decline from previous years.[7] As of 2016, there were 15.5 million cancer survivors in the United States, with the number projected to grow to about 20.3 million by 2026.[6,8] Despite this good news, the burden of cancer and its treatment can leave lasting physical, psychosocial, and economic consequences for patients and families.[9]

Cancer-related cognitive impairment (CRCI) can be defined as the broad array of memory and attention problems that develop during and following cancer and cancer treatment. CRCI has been empirically investigated for over three decades.[10–14] The most common complaints include problems with "short-term" memory, working memory, word recall, lack of concentration, and inability to "multitask." Survivors reporting these problems rate them as moderate to severe in intensity in self-report measures of CRCI symptoms.[13–16] However, self-report data are usually not highly correlated with objective neuropsychological test scores[17–20] and in fact tend to correlate more strongly with measures of emotional distress (anxiety, depression) and fatigue.[17,20] It may be that self-report measures capture the broader psychological response to the experience of CRCI more than objective neuropsychological tests administered under controlled, clinical conditions.

With respect to research on the prevalence of CRCI using neuropsychological testing measures, general rates vary widely among both cross-sectional and longitudinal studies (8% to 75%).[13,16,19] The differences in rates are thought to be due primarily to three factors: (1) a lack of consensus among research investigators on the definition of impaired neuropsychological test performance; (2) different neuropsychological tests used within different studies; and (3) wide variations in the cancer treatments received by survivors who participated in the studies (e.g., differing single-agent or combined chemotherapy regimens depending on individual clinical need). The latter point also has contributed to the limited knowledge about what specific agents or combinations lead to cognitive impairment.[13,16,19] Taking all these points into consideration, the broad consensus of the research literature is that just under or about half of those going through cancer and cancer treatment may experience some form of memory and attention problem following—and often many years after—treatment.

Despite the variability in estimated rates of CRCI, the following five points are consistent results across studies that users of this manual should know:

1) Neuropsychological domains of verbal recall, verbal working memory, and psychomotor processing speed appear impaired for cancer survivors versus control groups. Control participants are usually individuals with the same disease (e.g., breast cancer or lymphoma) matched for demographic factors such as age, IQ, and education, who have no history of neurologic disease and receive only local radiotherapy or surgery, with or without systemic therapies such as hormonal therapy, but who do not receive chemotherapy. Healthy individuals without cancer or neurologic impairment history have also been used as controls.[21]

2) Depressive and anxiety symptoms do not appear to play a role in differences on neuropsychological performances between survivors and matched controls. These variables have been reasonably well controlled in this body of research.[13,19,22,23]

3) Cognitive impairments detected among chemotherapy recipients appear to be in the mild to moderate range. While most studies demonstrate statistically significant differences between survivors and controls, neuropsychological test performances for individuals with CRCI can often be in the normal range. Therefore, the cognitive problems may be subtle, and neuropsychological tests may not be sensitive enough to detect cognitive performance declines in situations where the demands of task performance increase.[13,16,19,24]

4) Although cognitive problems may be subtle, they can last well beyond treatment. Studies with both longitudinal and cross-sectional designs have detected cognitive impairment among survivors relative to controls at 1 to 2 years after treatment and at 5 to 10 years.[14,22,25] That being said, it does appear that some survivors who experience cognitive effects during treatment can experience improvements soon after treatment ends.[26] It is unknown which individuals remain at risk for latent or prolonged cognitive problems.

5) Finally, most individuals with CRCI have stable symptoms and generally do not develop progressive cognitive decline. That is, memory function does not appear to get worse over time such as the decline observed in Alzheimer's disease or progressive dementias.[27] However, older cancer survivors are now receiving more research attention, and factors such as certain genetic markers, frailty status, and advanced age may interact with treatment type (e.g., chemotherapy or hormonal therapy in breast cancer) and contribute to cognitive decline.[28]

Causes of CRCI

It is beyond the scope of this manual to detail all possible mechanisms of CRCI. Which types of cancer or cancer treatment specifically lead to persistent CRCI remains under scientific investigation. By way of history, Ahles and Saykin[29] first summarized and proposed a number of candidate mechanisms in 2007, some of which have been supported by subsequent study. The causes reviewed here are those thought to be most helpful in rounding out the Memory and Attention Adaptation Training (MAAT) clinician's basic understanding of the variety of mechanisms that can contribute to a cancer survivor's CRCI. Early CRCI research focused primarily on the cognitive effects among cancer survivors of non-CNS disease who were treated with chemotherapy. However, other factors such as immune system and inflammatory responses to cancer itself, radiation therapy effects, hormonal changes, stem cell transplantation, and newer immunotherapies have also been found to affect cognitive function.[16] While the terms "chemobrain" or "chemofog" have become synonymous in describing CRCI, much has been learned in the past three decades suggesting that chemotherapy is not the only culprit.

Chemotherapies

While CRCI causes are multiple, MAAT clinicians should be familiar with the various types of chemotherapies and the research examining the relationship between chemotherapy and cognitive dysfunction. Having this basic understanding can facilitate better understanding of survivor experience and aid MAAT delivery. Table I.1 provides a brief overview of different classes of chemotherapy, how they generally work, some common side effects, and generic and brand names of examples. For a complete and updated reference source for chemotherapies, as well as a host of other cancer treatments, including immunotherapies, hormonal treatments, radiotherapies, and surgeries, refer to the website offered by Winship Cancer Institute at Emory University at https://www.cancerquest.org/patients/treatments.

"Cytotoxic" refers to drugs that kill rapidly growing cells. Cytotoxic chemotherapies are often given in combinations. For example, cyclophosphamide, methotrexate, and 5-fluorouracil are often combined (CMF), and data suggest greater cognitive dysfunction among patients receiving these drugs versus other chemotherapies such as anthracycline-containing regimens (including doxorubicin, epirubicin, and mitoxantrone), which are antibiotics used to treat various cancers.[30,31] However, the anthracyclines can present their own host of side effects, such as heart failure in some patients, and cardiac problems can also contribute to cognitive problems.[31] More research is needed to sort out which chemotherapy regimens are directly implicated in cognitive change.

It was once believed most chemotherapy agents did not cross the blood–brain barrier. However, research over the years has indicated that some agents do cross the blood–brain barrier and exert effects directly on neurons involved in memory function.[32-34] For example, positron emission tomography (PET) studies have found radiolabeled cisplatin in the brain at low concentrations after intravenous infusion. Even at these low concentrations, animal studies demonstrate cell death

Table I.1 Common Chemotherapies, Actions, and Side Effects

Classes of Chemotherapy	Common Drugs in Class (Generic and Brand Names)	Anti-Cancer Action	Side Effects	Cognitive Effects
Alkylating agents	cyclophosphamide (Cytoxan) ifosfamide (Ifex) cisplatin (platinum analog [Platinol])	Cause cell death by interacting with DNA during cell synthesis	Nausea, anemia	Suspected: cyclophosphamide ifosfamide
Anthracyclines	doxorubicin (Adriamycin) epirubicin (Ellence) mitoxantrone	Cytotoxic antibiotic (kills rapidly growing cells, non–cell-cycle-specific agents)	Toxicity to heart (arrhythmias), fever, hair loss, oral ulcers, white and red blood cell suppression	Suspected: doxorubicin, epirubicin
Taxanes	docetaxel (Taxotere) paclitaxel (Taxol)	Cytotoxic agents that disrupt tubulin, a protein needed for cell division	Hair loss, mouth sores, nausea, diarrhea, anaphylactic reactions, neutropenia	Suspected: docetaxel paclitaxel
Vinca alkaloids	vinblastine (Velban) vincristine (Oncovin) vinorelbine (Navelbine)	Act on M cell-cycle phase; another anti-tubulin agent that causes cell death; for both blood cancers (hematologic) and solid tumors	Nausea, hair loss, mouth sores, constipation, headache Bone marrow suppression with vinblastine	Unknown
Antimetabolites	methotrexate (Folex) fluorouracil (5-FU; Adrucil; Fluoroplex) gemcitabine (Gemzar) cytarabine (ara-C)	Molecules "mimic" cell protein that prevents normal binding of proteins, causing cell death (apoptosis)	Bone marrow suppression, anemia, bleeding, increased infection risk, nausea, diarrhea	Suspected: methotrexate fluorouracil cytarabine

and decreased cell division in the dentate gyrus of the hippocampus and corpus callosum,[35] regions important to memory function.

Genetic Vulnerabilities

To complicate matters, genetic vulnerabilities can modulate the extent to which chemotherapies can cross the blood–brain barrier and thus influence cognitive function. For instance, the gene multidrug resistance 1 (MDR1) encodes a protein, P-glycoprotein (P-gp), which plays a role in transporting toxic substances out of cells. P-gp influences drug uptake at the blood–brain barrier.[29] MDR1 variability in the population might explain in part some of the individual differences in cognitive function observed among survivors who receive the same chemotherapy and who have the same disease.

Other genetic markers have been investigated for their role in CRCI development and to help account for why some cancer survivors may be more vulnerable than others. The apolipoprotein E (APOE) ε4 allele has been found to play a role in neural repair and plasticity after brain injury. One study of long-term cancer survivors found that ε4 carriers scored significantly lower in visual-spatial abilities than non-ε4 carriers.[36] Also, APOE ε4 carriers, as opposed to carriers of other forms of APOE alleles, have been found to have morphological variations such as changes in gray matter[37] and decreased hippocampal volume.[38] However, some research on APOE ε4 carriers with cancer has found no relationship with cognitive change.[39] Therefore, there is no definitive evidence that all carriers of APOE ε4 will demonstrate cognitive change after cancer or cancer treatment.

Genetic polymorphisms associated with disruption of memory-related neurotransmission represent another area of scientific investigation. For example, catechol-O-methyl transferase (COMT) is an enzyme that has been associated with dopamine degradation in the frontal lobes and reduced cognitive function.[40] One study by Small et al.[41] examined the association between breast cancer survivors who were positive for the COMT valine allele (or COMT-Val+ allele) and neuropsychological test performance. COMT-Val+ individuals have been demonstrated to have more rapid degradation of frontal lobe dopamine transmission. COMT-Val+ survivors were hypothesized to have poorer neuropsychological test performance than those without this marker. The investigators confirmed these predictions. COMT-Val+ breast cancer survivors who received chemotherapy performed worse on neuropsychological tests of attention, verbal fluency, and motor speed than the breast cancer survivors who were not COMT-Val+. Moreover, COMT Val+ survivors performed worse than COMT-Val+ healthy controls. This suggests that, for some individuals, it is the interaction of genetic vulnerability (in this case COMT-Val+), cancer, and chemotherapy that leads to the development of CRCI.

The notion that non-CNS cancer itself can lead to CRCI has also been studied. Brain-derived neurotrophic factor (BDNF) is a protein that is encoded by the BDNF gene and is associated with neuron repair and neurogenesis. BDNF is expressed in the cerebral cortex and hippocampus. One animal study has shown that non-CNS tumors may induce hippocampal dysfunction through reducing BDNF availability and, hence, neurogenesis.[42] In other research, a BDNF polymorphism has been associated with poorer performance on measures of memory and executive function as well as lower hippocampal volume in a non-cancer sample.[43] It may be that some survivors—for example, those with BDNF genetic polymorphisms—may be more vulnerable to CRCI when they develop cancer due to potential alterations in BDNF. Investigation of the effects of BDNF polymorphisms and tumor-related BDNF alteration among cancer patients is ongoing.

Vascular Damage and Inflammation

Aside from genetic vulnerabilities, CRCI mechanisms having to do with changes in the brain's vascular system and immune responses have been studied. Microvascular damage and ischemic effects (i.e., "leaky" blood vessels) have been associated with cognitive impairment among cancer survivors.[33] Vascular endothelial growth factor receptor (VEGFR) tyrosine kinase inhibitors (or VEGFR TKIs) are drugs that have demonstrated much success in the treatment of renal cell carcinoma[44] and gastrointestinal stromal tumor (GIST).[45] VEGF plays important roles in CNS biology through angiogenesis and neurogenesis and is believed to be important for hippocampal function.[46] VEGFR TKIs have also been associated with lower neuropsychological test performance in 56 survivors of renal cell carcinoma and 4 patients with GIST compared with healthy controls.[47] This suggests that certain TKI therapies could alter hippocampal blood supply, thereby affecting cognitive function.

The role of pro-inflammatory cytokines has garnered much attention in CRCI research. Pro-inflammatory cytokines are proteins that play a role in immunity to help ward off disease by directing movement of immune system cells to infection or trauma. However, in larger numbers they may disrupt cell function and, for example, disrupt the health of neurons used in memory.[48,49] Elevated cytokine levels have been detected in breast cancer patients prior to treatment compared to healthy controls.[48] This suggests that the presence of cancer can lead to elevation of cytokine levels, then subsequent cognitive change.

In a similar process, some cancer therapies can trigger immune and inflammatory responses. For example, cognitive impairment has been observed in a number of patients with multiple myeloma (MM) who undergo autologous hematopoietic stem cell transplant (HSCT).[50] HSCT involves removal of a patient's healthy, preformed (stem) blood cells from the bone marrow (where certain blood cells are developed), storing the cells and incubating them with antibodies, then eradicating the patient's unhealthy, malignant cells with high-dose chemotherapy or radiation therapy, and finally "transplanting" or re-introducing the patient's stored cells. The re-introduction of the healthy cells may trigger a cytokine response that may in some cases lead to cognitive problems in the acute phase of recovery. Typically, some cognitive decline, then recovery, is seen over several weeks to months after the transplant.[50] In general, it may be this acute post-transplant response that has led to a fairly consistent finding that patients with hematologic malignancy who undergo HSCT are more likely to experience CRCI compared to non-cancer controls.[51] However, at least one study has shown that about 40% of participants had impairments at one year post-transplant.[52] Moreover, similar to observations made with breast cancer survivors, impairments have been observed in some patients with hematologic malignancies prior to HSCT.[53] There may be inflammatory responses bother before and after HSCT. Recent evidence suggests that patients undergoing HSCT have produced higher levels of inflammatory biomarkers of interleukin-6 (IL-6) and tumor necrosis factor (TNF).[54] Therefore, it may be likely that the combined inflammatory effects of disease and subsequent cancer treatment influence the development of CRCI in patients with hematologic cancers.

Hormonal and Endocrine Disruption

In the case of breast cancer, about 75% of cases are promoted by estrogen.[55] Hormonal therapies such as tamoxifen (a selective estrogen receptor modulator [SERM]) and anastrozole (an aromatase inhibitor [AI]) are designed to reduce estrogen availability and, in turn, reduce risk of breast cancer recurrence. However, estrogen also plays a role in verbal memory, and both SERMs and AIs have been shown to reduce verbal memory neuropsychological test performance.[56] SERMs and AIs are typically administered after surgery and/or chemotherapy and are often prescribed for 5 to 10 years. Therefore, for some breast cancer survivors, there is a balancing act between the benefits of recurrence risk reduction with these medicines versus the experience of mild to moderate impairments in memory and attention.[57]

Another hormonal cancer treatment, androgen deprivation therapy (ADT) for men with prostate cancer, may also adversely affect cognitive performance through testosterone reduction.[58,59] ADT treatment can last for 6 months for men who have an intermediate risk of advancing disease but up to 18 to 24 months for men who are at high risk (see https://www.cancer.gov/types/prostate/prostate-hormone-therapy-fact-sheet). More research on long-term effects of ADT and factors that can make men with prostate cancer more or less vulnerable to CRCI is ongoing. Among men with testicular cancer, there is evidence of cognitive decline in long-term survivors, but much of the CRCI research focus has been on cisplatin-based chemotherapies,[60] with less research on hormonal disruption. Research on men with testicular cancer has also shown that a confluence of factors, including treatment (chemotherapy, radiation therapy), pro-inflammatory cytokine activity, and genotype (APOE), can interact to produce CRCI. Reductions in neuropsychological test performance have also been associated with changes in the brain, including gray matter density as assessed by voxel-based morphometry and other imaging methods.[37] Again, it appears from much of the CRCI research to date that an interaction of variables having to do with genetics, treatment, and immune response to cancer itself produces cognitive change. As hinted here, there are underlying changes in brain structure and function that may help identify the complex mechanisms that underlie CRCI.

Brain Imaging and CRCI

There seem to be some common findings as to how the brain *responds and adapts to* cancer and cancer treatment. Over the years of CRCI research, neuropsychological test outcomes demonstrate mild or moderate change in test scores, usually with samples of people with high cognitive function before cancer. As a result, individual survivors who are evaluated for CRCI well after completion of active cancer treatment may report a high amount of cognitive symptoms in standardized self-report measures—but with neuropsychological test scores often falling within the normal range.[16,27] This presentation has fueled debate as to whether survivors who report CRCI have impairments that warrant treatment. However, data from brain imaging studies demonstrate differences in brain activation patterns during memory tasks between cancer survivors and those with no cancer history (with the groups matched on factors such as age, education, and IQ). This suggests that biological changes attributable to cancer and cancer therapies can account for mild or moderate cognitive impairments while the brain is under demand for cognitive performance.

In one early, small brain imaging study, Silverman et al.[25] used positron emission tomography (PET) to determine if there were differences between chemotherapy recipients and non-chemotherapy recipients in brain metabolism during cognitive tasks. The researchers compared 16 breast cancer survivors, 5 to 10 years after completion of chemotherapy (11 also had hormonal treatment [tamoxifen] following chemotherapy), to a small group ($n = 8$) of matched controls, some of whom had a breast cancer history but none of whom received chemotherapy. Each participant completed a short-term memory task while in the scanner. PET images demonstrated altered patterns in the frontal cortex, cerebellum, and basal ganglia among the chemotherapy recipients relative to the control participants. Task-related increases in prefrontal cortical blood flow were significantly greater for chemotherapy-exposed participants, suggesting these regions had increased metabolic activity to complete a memory task identical to that performed by controls. The investigators concluded that additional activation of the cortex and other brain regions represents a brain mechanism that compensates for chemotherapy-damaged regions through reorganized circuitry.

An intriguing case study of identical twins published by the first author and colleagues may point to more evidence of a cortical compensatory mechanism at play among individuals treated with chemotherapy.[61] This study involved 60-year-old female monozygotic twins who were both positive for the APOE ε4 allele (as discussed earlier, a genetic vulnerability for CRCI). One twin was diagnosed with breast cancer and received chemotherapy, while the other had no cancer history. Both were evaluated with a brief battery of neuropsychological tests and self-report measures of cognitive function and completed a visual vigilance and working memory task (the n-back task) while undergoing functional magnetic resonance imaging (fMRI).

Results showed the women performed comparably on neuropsychological testing and the n-back task. However, as seen in Figure I.1, the twin who underwent chemotherapy (top image) demonstrated more cortical activation as evidenced by more light and dark gray patches. Going from left to right, the n-back task becomes more difficult. By contrast, the unaffected twin (bottom image) did not produce as much activation as her sister who received chemotherapy. Both twins demonstrated more

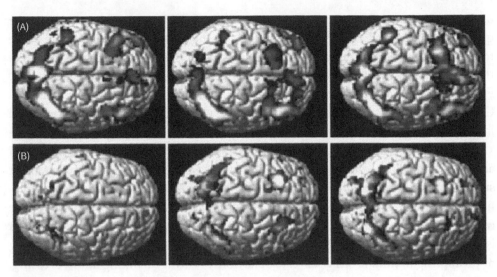

Figure I.1 fMRI images of twins doing a memory task that gets more difficult from left to right. Note that the twin who received chemotherapy (**A**) appears to have more activation of the brain for the same task than her non-cancer twin (**B**).

activation moving left to right with increasing task difficulty. This was expected, but the chemotherapy twin demonstrated broader activation. Moreover, the twin who received chemotherapy reported more difficulty with cognitive tasks than her unaffected sister on the Multiple Abilities Self-Report Questionnaire (MASQ), a self-report measure of daily cognitive failures.

While not conclusive, this case study does raise the possibility of a neural compensatory mechanism that may underlie cognitive complaints among some cancer survivors. It may also help explain why many individuals after cancer or chemotherapy can have normal performance or mild decline on neuropsychological testing but report they are "working harder" or are slower to achieve the same cognitive performance they were accustomed to prior to cancer. Subsequent imaging research has largely replicated and found the cortical compensatory mechanism in groups of breast cancer survivors, adding support to this hypothesis.[62,63] "Hyperconnectivity" has also been found in long-term survivors (>14 years after treatment) of testicular cancer who underwent cisplatin-based chemotherapy.[64] This brief twin study is summarized in the MAAT survivor workbook and is often a point of discussion in Visit 1.

Summary

Many candidate mechanisms are currently the focus of ongoing study on how cancer and cancer treatments adversely affect cognitive function. It is not critical to know each in detail, and reviewing each mechanism with individual survivors is neither necessary nor advised. However, having a basic understanding will be helpful background knowledge as you work with survivors. This section may help answer questions some survivors may have and, if nothing else, may help survivors come to appreciate the tremendous complexity of the problem as researchers continue their work. A good summary for clinicians can be found in a recent book chapter by Ferguson et al.,[16] and updated summaries are usually published by the International Cognition and Cancer Task Force (ICCTF; www.icctf.com) in peer-reviewed journals. ICCTF holds scientific conferences every two years.

In this section we did not cover research on all mechanisms associated with CRCI and, thus, not all potential types of CRCI survivors who may present. However, most survivors can likely benefit from MAAT, although MAAT research has focused primarily on chemotherapy recipients. Adults who have had CNS disease or who have had surgical excision can likely benefit from MAAT so long as cognitive dysfunction is not severe (defined as individuals who require supervision or who require cueing or prompting to initiate basic self-care behaviors of eating, drinking fluids, dressing, or bathing). Those with severe cognitive impairments as assessed by neuropsychological testing will require more intensive rehabilitative efforts than MAAT.

Problems with memory and attention can develop during cancer onset or during treatment and may linger well after treatment concludes. Cognitive functions are critical to complex behaviors of daily life. Planning, goal setting, task organization, and follow-through at home, the workplace, or school depend on cognitive performance. Much of the content in this introduction has reviewed the cognitive effects of cancer and its treatments, and it is intended as a brief summary and by no means is an exhaustive review of CRCI scientific knowledge. Regardless of the multiple etiologies of CRCI, MAAT can be used by clinicians as a cognitive-behavioral therapy (CBT) to aid improvement in each survivor's daily task performance and quality of life.

Background of MAAT

Prevention and treatment are key pursuits for research on any health problem. There are currently no known prophylactic or protective methods available prior to cancer treatment that may help prevent or reduce CRCI. There are some drug treatments that have been attempted following chemotherapy (such as dexmethylphenidate [Focalin]),[65] but without sound understanding of the neurobiological mechanisms at play, specific, targeted pharmacological therapies have not been developed. Further, many cancer survivors appear to prefer a non-drug approach after taking numerous drugs for cancer treatment that have aversive side effects. Indeed, in the Lower et al. study alone, 40.8% of participants reported headache and 27.6% reported nausea with dexmethylphenidate.[65] As more individuals are being diagnosed with cancer, many will likely experience CRCI whether it is related to needed life-saving treatment or cancer itself. Given our current knowledge of the problem and thus lack of targeted pharmacological therapies, it makes sense to develop, evaluate, and disseminate a brief, non-drug, psychological treatment option. MAAT is intended to fill this void.

MAAT utilizes cognitive-behavioral methods drawn from research on stress, anxiety, and symptom management in behavioral medicine and from various treatment approaches in cognitive rehabilitation. MAAT is designed to help individuals make adaptive changes to compensate for long-term memory dysfunction in daily life. This is in contrast to trying to improve the specific cognitive processes damaged, as with many traditional cognitive rehabilitation approaches. This "compensatory strategy approach" is based on the assumption that the individual will use retained cognitive functions to develop new adaptive behaviors to complete complex daily tasks that involve memory.[66,67] Specifically, MAAT aims to use a CBT approach to improve self-management of the impact of cognitive dysfunction in daily life—*to aid performance in valued tasks that require attention and memory, not to improve memory function in hopes that it generalizes or "transfers" to daily life tasks.* In this sense, MAAT's primary aim is to foster learning of *adaptive* behavior among those with CRCI.

Who Can Benefit from MAAT?

MAAT was developed primarily for individuals who have memory and attention problems following diagnosis of and treatment for cancer. Three studies evaluating the feasibility and efficacy of MAAT were conducted with breast cancer survivors.[61,68,69] In a fourth clinical trial MAAT was evaluated with either methylphenidate or placebo versus "behavioral placebo" among individuals with mild to moderate traumatic brain injury (MTBI).[70] However, in the clinical setting, cancer survivors with cancers other than breast cancer can likely benefit. This includes individuals who have had CNS disease or treatments such intracranial or whole-body irradiation, intrathecal therapies, androgen (hormonal) therapies for prostate cancer, stem cell transplantation, or surgical excision of brain tumors. In short, *the etiology of the cognitive complaints is not of primary concern.* That being said, for individuals with more severe cognitive impairments, such as those who require supervision or have a concurrent progressive dementia and lack awareness of their impairments, MAAT is unlikely to be helpful. They likely require more intensive and lengthy cognitive rehabilitation.

Theoretical Foundations of MAAT: An Adaptive Approach

Regardless of the neurologic source of cognitive problems, cancer survivors can likely compensate for memory and attention problems if they learn specific, adaptive behavioral strategies. The compensatory strategy approach has been found

to generalize (or "transfer") across multiple settings better than repetitive practice (computerized) interventions that limit improvement to trained tasks.[66,71-75]
A deeper theoretical understanding of MAAT is based on a diathesis-stress model
and social learning theory. This model (Figure I.2) takes into account the biological, complex etiological factors (e.g., cancer, chemotherapy, or other treatment exposure) that spawn CRCI and the multiple biopsychosocial factors that maintain it
and diminish quality of life.

Memory and attention are affected by multiple interacting neurocognitive systems. Affective states, physiological arousal, sensory acuity (i.e., hearing and seeing),
and environment all influence orientation, attention, encoding, speed of processing,
recognition, retrieval, and recall. Under routine, low-demand conditions, these
interacting neurocognitive systems function well. By contrast, under conditions
of increased demand, cognitive failures may be more frequent and produce negative consequences. MAAT, therefore, in part, assumes a diathesis-stress model
where CRCI-influenced cognitive systems are vulnerable under greater task difficulty (second box from top, right-hand side, Figure I.2). It is at this point where
the survivor experiences a perception of disparity between "perceived threat level"
(memory demand) and available resources to effectively contend with the demand
(lowered perceived cognitive abilities). This leads to increased arousal, distress, and,
in turn, reduced cognitive performance. This perceived disparity between threat and

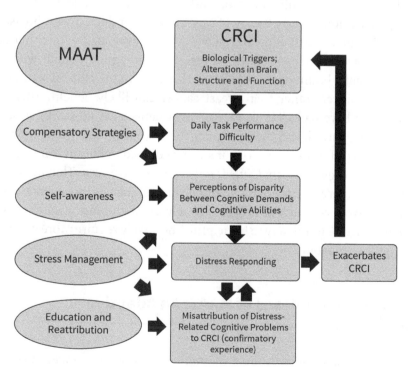

Figure I.2 Diathesis-stress and appraisal model of CRCI and MAAT components of change

resource availability is based on the Lazarus[76] two-step appraisal model of stress, where threat perceptions alone are not sufficient to trigger stress responses unless accompanied by perceptions of inadequate personal or external resources to meet the threat. In this model, "diatheses" are vulnerabilities in cognitive function produced by the survivor's cancer and/or treatment exposure (e.g., chemotherapy, brain structural/functional changes) as well as other factors such as pre-cancer neurocognitive status, education,[14] age,[14] genetic predispositions, cognitive reserve,[14,77] and emotional resilience.[14,78] The more a cancer survivor with CRCI can train and make effortful, efficient use of existing cognitive capacities *and* learn and apply new skills, the greater the cognitive task performance, perception of increased control over memory performance (to meet demands), and consequent distress reduction (Figure I.2).

MAAT's central aim is to build adaptive skills and mastery experience to reduce disparity between perceived coping resources and cognitive demands. With increased mastery experience with cognitive tasks, survivors begin to make more attributions of memory performance to controllable factors, such as attentive effort, versus uncontrollable causes of cancer and cancer treatment exposure. This "reattributional" shift to controllable causes of memory performance builds motivation for survivors to engage in and persist with more cognitively demanding activity,[79,80] experience more mastery with memory tasks, and reduce distress (Figure I.2).[79,81,82] In sum, MAAT aims to help individuals acquire compensatory memory and adaptive behavioral coping skills to perform better at daily functional tasks—as rehabilitation expert Dr. Barbara Wilson has said, "tasks for which memory is used."[67]

MAAT Research

Investigation of MAAT efficacy is ongoing, but several studies have been completed supporting efficacy. In the first study, MAAT was pilot-tested for feasibility and to determine if it could positively influence daily cognitive symptoms, neurocognitive test performance, and quality of life. In a single-arm study,[61] 29 breast cancer survivors (mean 8.2 years post-chemotherapy) reporting cognitive problems completed MAAT. Principal outcome measures included the MASQ (self-report of cognitive function in daily life),[83] the Quality of Life–Cancer Survivors scale (QOL-CS),[84] satisfaction ratings, and a brief neurocognitive test battery administered at baseline, post-treatment, and the two-month and six-month follow-ups. Results indicated significant reductions in daily cognitive complaints, improved quality of life, and high satisfaction. Neurocognitive improvements in verbal episodic memory and processing speed were also observed. However, with no control group, it was impossible to rule out effects of practice with repeat neurocognitive testing.

The second MAAT study was a small waitlist (no treatment) control randomized controlled trial (RCT).[68] Forty breast cancer survivors who were at least 18 months post-chemotherapy and who were reporting cognitive problems were randomized to MAAT ($n = 19$) or waitlist control ($n = 21$) conditions and assessed at baseline, post-treatment, and the two-month follow-up. Controlling for education and IQ, MAAT participants made significant improvements over waitlist participants on quality of life and episodic memory as assessed by the California Verbal Learning Test-II (CVLT-II). Subtracting waitlist control effects, the pre-to-post-treatment effect size (Cohen's *d*) for the CVLT-II total score was −0.50 and quality-of-life effect size was −0.49 (note that the negative sign does not change the magnitude of the effect). CVLT-II scores for MAAT participants also improved at the two-month follow-up ($d = -0.63$).

In the third MAAT trial, an active control condition (supportive therapy [ST]) was added.[69] ST is a common active control condition in CBT trials to control for psychological therapy "common factors" such as interpersonal warmth, empathy, and treatment expectation. Outcome measures were improved with the addition of the self-report measure Functional Assessment of Cancer Therapy–Cognitive scale (FACT-Cog).[85] Both MAAT and ST were delivered via videoconference network linking rural health centers throughout Maine.[86] The primary aim of the study was to evaluate electronic delivery feasibility and efficacy. Adjusting for baseline differences, MAAT participants ($n = 35$) improved in FACT-Cog perceived cognitive impairments (PCI) over ST at the 2-month follow-up ($p = 0.02$; $d = 0.52$), and MAAT participants had a significant improvement in processing speed over controls at post-treatment ($p = 0.03$; $d = 0.50$), with continued sustained improvement over baseline at the two-month follow-up. Finally, MAAT participants had a trend ($p = 0.07$) for improvement over ST in anxiety about cognitive symptoms (Meta-Memory in Adulthood Anxiety Scale) with a large effect size ($d = 0.90$) at the two-month follow-up. This suggests that MAAT participants continued to make gains in reduced emotional distress about cognitive symptoms while ST participants regressed to baseline two months after cessation of therapeutic contact. Presumably, MAAT participants had acquired and mastered a skillset that would continue to be applied and improved despite no contact with their clinician, whereas those survivors in the ST arm did not. MAAT participants also reported they were highly likely to recommend treatment to a friend and indicated they likely would *not* have been able to participate without videoconference delivery. While promising, limitations of this study include small sample size and only one clinician delivering MAAT and one delivering ST. This trial also did not show the between-group difference in episodic memory (CVLT-II) seen in the waitlist control trial. In both trials, controls only made 2-point gains in CVLT-II score from baseline to the two-month follow-up, while MAAT participants made 8-point and 4-point gains in the waitlist and ST control trials, respectively. With a larger RCT and thus higher statistical power, it seems likely CVLT-II differences would emerge.

The fourth study evaluated MAAT efficacy in individuals with at least four months of persistent cognitive complaints or objective cognitive impairment following MTBI.[70] In a multi-site and multi-clinician RCT, MAAT was compared with an attention control repetitive practice intervention that was identical to MAAT in terms of time spent with the clinician ("Attention Builders Training" [ABT]) in a two-by-two design with or without pharmacological enhancement (methylphenidate [MPH] or placebo). Participants were randomized to one of four conditions: MAAT/MPH (n = 17), ABT/MPH (n = 19), MAAT/placebo (n = 17), or ABT/placebo (n = 18). Neurocognitive and self-report assessments were administered at baseline and after treatment. Linear regression models controlling for baseline score, study site, treatment adherence, and time since injury showed the following: MAAT/placebo > ABT/placebo for episodic memory (CVLT-2; p = 0.04); MAAT/MPH > ABT/MPH for auditory working memory (p = 0.02); and MAAT/MPH > MAAT/placebo and ABT/MPH for nonverbal learning (p = 0.02 and 0.03, respectively). Effect sizes (Cohen's d) ranged from 0.3 to 0.8. Results suggest MAAT, alone or in combination with MPH, can improve cognitive outcomes among individuals with prolonged TBI symptoms. In addition, fMRI, obtained in a subset of participants (~50%), showed greater working memory–related frontal activation during the n-back task (as used in the twin study cited earlier) for MAAT participants versus ABT participants. In addition, increased activation post-treatment showed a trend-level correlation with improved task performance.[87] This suggests that MAAT may enhance frontal systems activation, leading to neurocognitive improvement. More research with greater power to detect such effects could produce important evidence speaking to MAAT's mechanism of efficacy (e.g., engagement of frontal networks to support cognition).

The result of research to date on MAAT suggests that it is efficacious and can be delivered via telehealth services, or face to face, with no difference in clinical effectiveness.[68,69,88] MAAT emphasizes cognitive modification or restructuring by reviewing in detail the therapeutic benefit of "memory failure reattribution"—that is, helping survivors make important and careful distinctions between everyday memory failure due to the contributions of inattention, stress, and emotional arousal (factors more controllable) versus failures that are due solely to cancer or cancer treatment (factors less controllable). This is explained fully in the next section. The intent of memory failure reattribution is to minimize faulty causal attributions that can lead to emotional distress surrounding the aversive experience of cognitive symptoms. A brief section in Visit 3 on basic cognitive restructuring is presented to aid survivors in stress management using common evidence-based cognitive modification methods. These MAAT elements are based on the available evidence of MAAT effectiveness. Results to date have helped contribute to MAAT's development in an empirically guided way.

An Important Note on Real-World Clinical Presentation

CRCI research summarized in this manual has largely been conducted with carefully selected participants so that confounding factors such as previous brain injury,

CNS disease, pathological anxiety or depression, etc. did not confound conclusions. Clinical scientists had to rule out and control for the effects of these conditions, and, as a result, cancer survivors with these and similar problems who develop CRCI have largely gone unstudied. However, this raises an important question: What if individuals with preexisting brain injury or other conditions (such as anxiety disorders) are the most vulnerable to the cognitive effects of cancer or cancer treatment? With this in mind, MAAT can most likely be used with such individuals because it utilizes a compensatory-adaptive behavior change approach, provided that, a previous condition such as a mood or anxiety disorder is not severe enough to overwhelm the individual's ability to actively participate in MAAT.

Of course, the use of MAAT in clinical practice must be done only after thorough assessment. If anxiety or mood disorders or more profound psychiatric or neurologic conditions are present, the clinician must determine whether those problems should be addressed more intensely before undertaking MAAT. If the functional impact of these problems is significant, the individual should have those treated first so that they may get the most out of MAAT. Also, MAAT is intended as a brief CBT for mild cognitive impairment and not progressive cognitive decline such as conditions of advancing dementia. As seen in the following sections, MAAT does require some self-regulatory behaviors of basic planning, task identification, task initiation, and follow-through. Individuals with severely disordered behavior and cognition will likely not benefit.

Finally, "manualized" treatments such as MAAT come under criticism because they may lack flexibility and are not "self-correcting" in response to survivors' needs over the course of treatment. This does not have to be so. In clinical settings, MAAT can be shortened or lengthened (number of visits) with adjustments to the visit schedule. Again, MAAT will likely be most effective if pretreatment assessment identifies other problems that can interfere with the work required to make progress. Open discussion with each survivor about their willingness or time availability to commit to MAAT is encouraged. In the MAAT survivor workbook, there is a segment devoted to this topic. Survivors should be encouraged to look this over if they are unsure or can't decide if they want to start. This is all part of sound practice and treatment preparation. In summary, MAAT can be used flexibly and with survivors who present in the real world.

Treatment Plan

MAAT involves eight visits of 45 to 53 minutes each and can be done individually with a psychologist (or other health professional) or in small groups. Some visits may be 30 minutes in duration depending on the survivor's individual situation, preferences, and mastery of compensatory strategies. In each visit, survivors will learn skills and then will practice them at home between visits. "Practice" in MAAT really means the practical application of strategies in everyday, real-life situations.

For research purposes, visits should be completed on a weekly basis, although there is no reason why visits can't be held twice weekly or once every two to three weeks depending on survivor circumstances in clinic settings (e.g., distances from the cancer care facility, job schedule). It is also assumed with this CBT that consistent application of strategies in daily life is the most important element of treatment effectiveness, not the total time in face-to-face or videoconference contact with the treating clinician. In a previous version of MAAT, phone contacts between visits were part of the program to help reinforce survivors' efforts at applying compensatory strategies. There is no reason why in clinical settings phone contacts can't be used in this manner.

Each survivor will receive a MAAT survivor workbook with information about cancer-related problems of memory and attention, as well as simple, concise, step-by-step written guides on cognitive skills taught in individual visits. The clinician should read and review the survivor workbook. The clinician should also be well versed in all teaching procedures for the compensatory cognitive skills detailed in this manual. Survivors are asked to bring the workbook with them to *each visit* and to read relevant sections between visits, along with applying the learned compensatory strategies. Survivors are encouraged to ask questions and mark content in the workbook to clarify with the clinician. This treatment approach emphasizes collaboration between clinician and survivor to empower each cancer survivor to become his or her own "memory and attention clinician."

The Four Components of MAAT

MAAT consists of four cognitive-behavioral components that address the biopsychological factors that serve to create and maintain CRCI distress depicted in Figure I.2:

1) **Education and Reattribution**—emphasizing basics of memory and attention function, normal cognitive failure, and what is and is not known about CRCI.
2) **Self-awareness training**—emphasizing awareness of the multiple influences that affect experience of memory and attention failures, such as symptom expectations, environmental demands, stress, and chemotherapy and other cancer treatments.
3) **Self-regulation**—emphasizing arousal self-regulation and stress coping skills along with gradual resumption of previously avoided functional activity.
4) **Compensatory strategies**—skills training to facilitate optimal functioning despite cognitive dysfunction. Compensatory strategies are intended to enlist intact cognitive functions to "compensate" for cognitive functions that may be harmed by cancer or cancer treatment. The intent is to use compensatory strategies to attain desired task performance despite cognitive problems. Compensatory strategies are divided into two subtypes: internal strategies and

external strategies, as conceptualized by Robin West, Ph.D., professor emer-
itus of aging and memory at the University of Florida,[89] and a term used by
other cognitive rehabilitation experts.[90,91] Internal strategies are methods
that are covert, such as cognitive and mnemonic strategies— "internal" to the
person. This may include verbal rehearsal, such as repeating something until it
becomes encoded information. External strategies refer to environmental cues
or use of devices "external" to the person (e.g., visual cues such as sticky notes,
paper or electronic calendars, or using a mobile phone to take a photo of where
the car is parked).

An outline of the treatment protocol is seen in Table 1.1 in Visit 1 of this manual. The
brief treatment format was selected as being the most feasible for integration within
a comprehensive or community cancer center, oncology service, or other medical
care setting where cancer survivors are seen. To use a traditional CBT format of 12
to 20 visits of 50 or more minutes each would likely consume high amounts of scarce
clinician time and clinic resources and would limit the number of cancer survivors
seen, leading to a growing waitlist. Other brief behavioral treatments have long
been successfully integrated in other medical settings and have demonstrated efficacy.[92] Previous outcome data from CBT for individuals with attention and memory
problems due to persistent MTBI symptoms (e.g., post-concussion syndrome)
suggest that cognitive symptom intensity is reduced after five clinician contacts.[93]
Therefore, some individuals going through MAAT may find beneficial change in
fewer than eight visits with minimal contact.

Telehealth and MAAT

Videoconference or telehealth delivery of MAAT is strongly encouraged. As
cited previously, the randomized trial of MAAT delivered via videoconferencing
demonstrated positive outcomes. Many cancer survivors, especially those who are of
working age, will have used limited leave time from their employers in order to meet
the rigorous schedules of cancer treatment, oncology follow-up appointments, and
numerous imaging and laboratory visits. Many have traveled great distances to get to
cancer care and struggled significantly to resume the pre-cancer vocational roles and
roles within their families or communities. Taking valuable time away from family,
work, or important life tasks is either too costly or just not an option in the recovery
from active cancer treatment. Telehealth technology has provided a tremendous opportunity to expand care access for survivors and minimize time and travel burdens.
It has also provided a means of keeping cancer survivors safe during the global
pandemic of COVID-19 of 2020. In the aforementioned videoconference trial,
participants utilized videoconferencing that allowed them to participate in MAAT,
but due to both technological and regulatory conditions, they were still required to
travel to a local medical facility that had videoconference devices. At the time of this

writing, software technology fortunately allows secure, encrypted connections directly to survivors' homes or other private settings using mobile device technology. The lead author uses this technology for delivery of MAAT to both urban and rural survivors from the University of Pittsburgh Medical Center, Hillman Cancer Center, and outcomes are positive with survivors of varying forms of cancer and varying degrees of survivorship complications (e.g., anxiety, chronic fatigue, or neuropathic pain). Cancer centers, health care settings, and private psychology practices are rapidly increasing telehealth services, and thus MAAT may be more readily available to survivors who might otherwise not have access. That said, technological and regulatory matters (such as privacy or practice jurisdiction) are not fully resolved and are ever evolving.[94] Therefore, using MAAT through these modalities should be done with care and with sound knowledge of national and local telehealth law and practice guidelines.[95,96] Getting the proper training, supervision, and continuing education to utilize telehealth technology prior to implementation is advised.

Using This Manual in Practice

In the following chapters, each of the eight MAAT visits are described. Before seeing any survivor, read this manual in its entirety and be familiar with the content covered in each visit.

Review the key points in each visit. Each key point is blocked in small bulleted paragraphs for simplicity and clarity to aid clinician learning. This treatment manual is not to be used or read from during visits, as emphasized earlier in the introduction. Rather, copy or print the Agenda and Clinician's Checklist at the head of each visit section and place it on a clipboard to help you keep track during the visit.

Visit 1

Agenda and Clinician Checklist

1. *Introduction and MAAT Overview*
___ Name of MAAT, brief rationale, provide workbook.
___ Review of MAAT schedule (Table 1.1).
2. *Education on Memory and Attention Effects of Cancer and Cancer Treatments*
___ Roughly up to half of individuals with cancer or following treatment can experience subtle attention and memory difficulty.
___ Not everyone is affected, but those who are tend to have verbal memory and executive function problems (working memory, processing speed).
___ This can be long-lasting (years) but not progressive (not worse with time).
___ Causes are unclear, but changes in brain chemistry (chemotherapy, anti-estrogen effects of hormonal therapy), micro-blood vessel damage, and potential genetic vulnerability (APOE) are identified contributors, but more study is needed.
___ Bottom line: About half of cancer survivors may demonstrate long-term memory complaints; the exact prevalence remains unclear and causes are unknown, but compensatory strategies can lessen the negative impact on daily life.
3. *Memory Failure Reattribution: Not All Memory Failures Are Cancer-Related*
___ Common cancer-related memory problems (Table 1.2)—Ask, "do any of these match your experience?" Allow survivor to discuss experience with cognitive problems.
___ Now compare/contrast common memory problems of everyday life (Table 1.3).
___ Memory and attention failures are common, but not all are attributable to cancer, though clearly many can be.
___ **Important rationale**—Since we don't know all the causes of cancer-related memory problems, we know that factors such as stress (physiological changes), fatigue, and divided attention of busy, daily life also contribute to memory problems.
___ We can change environment, alter stress response, manage fatigue, and use compensatory strategies to minimize effects of memory failures.
___ Focus is on improving current cognitive function, not on what is "lost."
4. *Self-Awareness and Monitoring Memory Problems*
___ Rationale: Identify environmental, affective, cognitive antecedents of memory failures in daily life ("know your 'at risk' situations").

___ Instruction for completion.

___ Not every memory failure is recorded but a sample of four or five forms for Visit 2.

5. *Progressive Muscle Relaxation (PMR)*

___ Rationale: Reduce sympathetic arousal that interferes with attention, encoding, and recall.

___ Enhance awareness of letting go of muscle tension *all the time, not just when stressed, to cultivate a lower baseline of arousal.*

___ Instructions: Flex muscles when you hear the word "now"—gentle flex, 30%.

___ Allow muscles to "drop" when told to relax.

___ Ignore the flexing command if a body part hurts—just focus on relaxing the muscle.

___ Instruct for home practice with audio recording.

6. *Homework*

___ Read MAAT workbook introduction and Visit 1—reassure it is all there.

___ Complete self-monitoring.

___ Daily PMR with audio recording.

Therapeutic Note

At the beginning of MAAT you will provide the treatment overview, rationale, and course to the survivor. This is a didactic approach. However, try to be as interactive as possible by asking questions to clarify concepts; invite survivors to share their experiences and thoughts about topics presented. Often, survivors will relate personal experience with cancer treatment to one or several concepts presented in Visit 1. This approach, combined with Socratic questioning methods, helps lead survivors to conclusions about the concepts presented. This will foster greater consolidation of learning and engender deeper concept understanding through active discovery.

An example of this therapeutic style is in presenting the finding that in general, most survivors who report cancer-related memory problems have difficulty with verbal memory. You might lead into this point with, *"What do you think is one of the most common types of memory problems reported by people who have had cancer?"* Regardless of the answer, you have now asked an open-ended question that creates a learning dialogue rather than a simple "yes" or "no" response. For example, if the survivor answers "remembering words, names, or things discussed in a conversation," the clinician may respond, *"Yes, in fact, verbal memory problems tend to be common in cancer-related memory problems, but memory problems with speed of processing occur as well. What is your experience?"* In sum, try not to dominate the discussion, but foster interaction. Many clinicians ask, "But how do I stay on topic and cover all the points if we engage in a lot of discussion?" In general, as you learn MAAT and gain experience, this becomes easier as you learn shorthand for concepts. You do not have to cover every single educational point about CRCI, but do cover those in the checklist—remember, survivors will have a workbook for reading and home review. Encourage survivors to ask questions at the following visit if one or more arise from reading. Also, it is helpful to tell survivors when introducing MAAT you may "reserve the right to compassionately interrupt" to help stay on track and manage time. When you see 15 minutes are left in the visit, simply say, "I'm mindful of the time," to cue the survivor that you will be wrapping up in 10 to 15 minutes to allow an adequate summary within the allotted timeframe. By and large, our experience tells us that the vast majority of survivors are eager to get on with the learning process and help keep the schedule.

Introduction and MAAT Overview

The name of this treatment program is Memory and Attention Adaptation Training. Emphasis is on adaptation, as we are fostering new learning to better compensate for memory problems in everyday life and minimize their impact.

- If not already done, provide the survivor with the workbook.
- The survivor can expect to learn:
  - The nature of memory and attention functions and how cancer can affect them.
  - Strategies to help better handle daily, real-world tasks that memory problems have affected; tasks at home, workplace, school, or social settings.
- Review the schedule of MAAT—weekly 45- to 50-minutes visits as outlined in Table 1.1.
- Remind the participant to bring the workbook to each visit.

Education on Memory and Attention and Effects of Cancer and Cancer Treatments

- Describe empirical findings summarized in the introduction section of this manual—these need not be covered in fine detail. Remember, engage participants in discussion and ask if findings math their experience. Points are bulleted as follows:
  - About half of individuals who have had cancer and undergo treatment may have measurable memory and attention problems. The real rate is unclear because of different ways of measuring and defining memory deficits.
  - Research suggests cancer-related memory and attention problems tend to be mild when measured by neuropsychological tests, but this can also vary among individuals.

Table 1.1 MAAT Schedule

Visit	Content
1	• Introduction and MAAT overview • Education on memory and attention and effects of cancer and treatment • Memory failure reattribution: Not all memory failures are cancer-related • Self-awareness and monitoring memory problems • Progressive muscle relaxation • Homework
2	• Review MAAT reading, relaxation and quick relaxation review, rehearsal • Review self-monitoring, effects of context, senses and memory problems • Internal strategy: Self-Instructional Training (SIT) • Homework
3	• Quick relaxation review • Review application of SIT • Internal strategy: verbal rehearsal strategies (verbal rehearsal, spaced rehearsal, chunking, and rhymes) • Cognitive restructuring: realistic probabilities and decatastrophizing • Homework
4	• Review of verbal rehearsal strategies • Review realistic probabilities and decatastrophizing • External strategy: keeping a schedule and memory routines • Homework
5	• Review of keeping a schedule and memory routines • External strategies: external cueing and distraction reduction • Activity scheduling and pacing • Homework
6	• Review of external cueing, distraction reduction, and activity scheduling and pacing • Internal and external strategy: active listening, verbal rehearsal for socializing • Fatigue management and sleep improvement • Homework
7	• Review active listening, verbal rehearsal for socializing • Review fatigue management and sleep quality improvement • Internal strategy: visualization strategies • Homework
8	• Review visualization strategies • Tying it together and continued quality-of-life improvement in survivorship • Discussion and wrap-up

• It is also known that anxiety, depression, and stress are not factors that produce impairments. Research has controlled for these problems and yet many survivors may still have mild cognitive change. That said, in clinical practice, depressive symptoms, major depressive disorder, and problematic anxiety and stress can certainly contribute to problems, so it is good to address these since more is known about them.

• Most survivors complain of memory problems during treatment and right after. By about six months many recover fully—but as already stated, some individuals have problems that persist a long time after treatment, even years.

• An online survey conducted by Hurricane Voices Breast Cancer Foundation found that 79% of 471 participants reported their cognitive symptoms had a gradual onset; 92% of 102 respondents reported their memory problems extended 5 years beyond the end of treatment.

- On the other hand, there is little evidence to suggest that survivors with persistent memory and attention problems after cancer get worse. CRCI is not dementia or a progressive illness such as Alzheimer's disease.

- Most research suggests problems with verbal memory, or memory for words, or things that were said. Deficits have also been observed in visual-spatial memory and processing speed.

- The exact causes of CRCI memory problems are unknown. As with many things in clinical science, the causal mechanisms are likely multiple. Mechanisms can include:

  - Estrogen suppression effects; estrogen is associated with verbal memory function. Menopause induced by chemotherapy or hormonal therapies such as tamoxifen or Arimidex (anastrozole) are known to contribute to mild verbal memory change.
  - Microvascular changes ("leaky" small blood vessels) related to chemotherapy.
  - Direct toxic effects of some chemotherapy drugs on neurons involved in memory. Methotrexate and cyclophosphamide can have these effects.
  - Genetic influences: The APOE (fourth allele) genetic marker is known to be associated with prolonged memory problems after coronary-artery bypass graft (CABG) surgery or after sport-related concussion. However, results among cancer survivors are mixed—not all individuals who are APOE positive develop memory problems after cancer and cancer therapy. COMT is also associated with prolonged memory problems among breast cancer survivors—however, more research on this factor is necessary.
  - Inflammation: The immune system in response to cancer can increase the release of pro-inflammatory cytokines, which can influence the hippocampus, a deep brain structure that processes and encodes memory.

- Bottom line: We know that just under or about half of cancer survivors can have memory and attention problems after cancer treatment. We do not know exactly what causes these problems, but there are likely a number of factors for any given individual. We do know some strategies can help people improve management of memory problems in general. That is what MAAT consists of: practical memory and attention strategies designed to improve cognitive skills the individual has, not focus on what is "lost."

Memory Failure Reattribution: Not All Memory Failures Are Cancer-Related

Outlining the rationale for the treatment is critical to:

- Enhance the collaborative nature of the clinician–participant relationship.
- Foster success in working toward a common goal of learning and using cognitive compensatory strategies.

Rationale for this program:

- We do not fully understand the *causes* of cancer-related cognitive changes, but we do know that other factors such as stress, inattention, and dealing with the distractions of numerous daily tasks *contribute* to memory problems in daily life.
- Some strategies can help improve daily performance in tasks *for which memory is used*[67]—even if the causes of memory problems are unknown.

Therapeutic Note:

- Memory failure reattribution is perhaps *the most important point made in MAAT.* It lays the theoretical foundation for the rationale of treatment. Specifically, while there is evidence that cancer itself, adjuvant chemotherapy, or other cancer treatment can produce long-lasting mild to moderate cognitive dysfunction, it is also true that not all memory and attention failures of daily life can be avoided. In fact, "normal forgetting" or lapses in memory are critical for cognitive health and rests at the crux of executive functions to "sort out what is important, and what is not." Thus, the brain can more efficiently use its limited cerebral memory storage networks. For example, it is far more important for an information technology specialist to remember major features of a new software package than it is to know what he or she had for lunch last Tuesday.
- In short, helping the survivor understand and accept memory and attention failures of daily life is likely therapeutic, in that the survivor can make more adaptive causal attributions when daily memory failures arise. Rather than attributing all or many daily cognitive failures to the lingering effects of cancer or cancer treatment, the survivor will come to understand that other, inherently more controllable factors, such as stress, fatigue, and inattention, also contribute to memory failures. This sets the stage for changing helpless, distress-related cognition (e.g., "it's my chemobrain again; I can't do anything about this") to more adaptive problem-solving cognitions (e.g., "OK, I just forgot to do this. What was happening so I can use some strategy to help prevent or adjust to this problem?"). Again, it is not the case that causal attributions for cognitive symptoms account for CRCI, but misattributions of daily memory failure to the salient event of cancer or treatment may be a psychological factor that *maintains emotional distress with cognitive symptoms.* This process is depicted in Figure I.2 of the introduction and has been observed in post-concussion syndrome[97] and in recent research on small sample of cancer survivors.[98]
- In sum, the present reattribution section of MAAT is designed to put the survivor on a track of enhancing coping self-efficacy and make efforts to mitigate the effects of memory failures in daily life. This is the essential element of the compensatory strategy adaptive approach of MAAT.

In this part of the visit, show the survivor two tables. The first, Table 1.2 of this manual and the workbook, lists common CRCI complaints. Ask:

"Do any of these memory problems match your experience?"

Table 1.2 Common Attention and Memory Problems Reported by Cancer Survivors

1. Recalling names
2. Recalling things when trying hard
3. Recalling written details on a form
4. Recalling written information or things viewed on television
5. Remembering names, faces of people recently met
6. Making sense out of verbal explanations
7. Recalling what happened just a few minutes ago
8. Paying attention to what is going on in the immediate environment
9. Following what people are saying
10. Staying alert to what is going on

Allow the survivor to read through them and explain which ones occur and how and when they do. Allow time for the survivor to "tell the story" of their memory failure experiences. We have found that this step frequently offers the survivor a form of support that he or she is not alone. After some time spent on this, direct the survivor's attention to Table 1.3. This is a list of common memory problems experienced by individuals in the general public, presumably with no neurologic impairment or previous history of brain injury. Point out that this list of daily memory problems is highly similar to that of individuals who report cancer-related memory problems. The intent of this is *not to invalidate* the survivor's experience or dismiss their memory problems—chances are, they have already experienced invalidation with their CRCI complaints to this point. Rather, the intent here is to point out that although memory problems are known to occur in a number of cancer survivors well after treatment completion, *not all failures of memory or attention are due to cancer or cancer treatment.*

Table 1.3 Common Things People Forget

Problem	Percent of People
Forgets telephone numbers	58%
Forgets people's names	48%
Forgets where car was parked	32%
Loses car keys	31%
Forgets groceries	28%
Forgets why they entered a room	27%
Forgets directions	24%
Forgets appointment dates	20%
Forgets store locations in shopping center	20%
Loses items around the house	17%
Loses wallet or pocketbook	17%
Forgets content of daily conversations	17%

Source: Mittenberg W, Zielinski R, Fichera S. Recovery from mild head injury: A treatment manual for patients. *Psychotherapy in Private Practice* 1993;12:37–52.

You may make two points here. First, "normal forgetting" is part of cognitive health, and executive functions are designed to distinguish the important from the not so important (as we mentioned earlier). Second, stress, inattention due to distraction, fatigue, and being hungry can all affect memory and attention. Since we know there are strategies to deal with these factors, *which are controllable*, the compensatory skills in MAAT are designed to recapture some self-efficacy in managing CRCI symptoms. The focus of MAAT is on what is known to enhance performance on daily tasks *for which memory is used.*[67] Learning and applying practical strategies to daily situations where one is "at risk" of memory problems is the goal of MAAT.

Model dialogue:

"Now that we have reviewed some of the facts about cancer-related memory problems, let me draw your attention to this table [Table 1.2]. This is a 'top 10 list' of common memory and attention problems reported by cancer survivors. Do any of these match your experience?"

Allow reasonable time (within limits) for the survivor to comment and tell their story.

"Now let me draw your attention to another table [Table 1.3]. As you can see, this is similar to the last table. However, it lists memory and attention problems in daily life reported by people who have not had cancer or any known neurologic problem such as brain injury, stroke, learning disability, or other type of brain injury."

Allow time for the survivor to review and note similarities.

"Many of these reported problems are similar to complaints reported by cancer survivors." (You may note some of the findings, such as nearly half of healthy individuals report difficulty in remembering names.)

"Now I want to be clear: The point of showing you these two tables is not to say, 'See, your cancer memory problems [or cancer brain, chemobrain, or chemofog] are just like everyone else's memory problems!' We already know from findings discussed earlier that you may have more problems after your cancer diagnosis. However, we also know that not all memory and attention problems in daily life are due only to cancer. Many incidents of forgetting or lapses in attention have to do with normal functions of the brain. 'Normal forgetting' is one way that the brain's executive functions—or systems of organization—sort out what is important to remember and what is not."

Await comment and discuss. You may even describe "hyperthymesia" or "excessive remembering," an exceedingly rare condition where the individual remembers every life event in fine detail. While no two people are alike, some individuals with hyperthymesia experience being burdened with emotionally painful memory—such as recalling adolescent awkwardness—and have difficulty coping. An interesting article was published on this topic on the website of the Smithsonian Institute in 2012 (https://www.smithsonianmag.com/innovation/rare-people-who-remember-everything-24631448/).

"Another reason we are going over these two tables is to help change excessive stress responses when memory problems come up. They may certainly be upsetting. But by understanding that other factors such as normal forgetting, stress, inattention, hunger, or fatigue can all contribute to memory problems, this can help start the focus on things we can change. It is important to recognize that even a frustrating thought such as, 'Oh, my cancer [or chemo] brain is back' can trigger a change in brain blood flow, taking away blood flow and resources from memory and recall functions and sending them to sensory areas of sight and sound to scan for danger. Similar to a deer that is startled when it hears a noise or sees a person in the woods. It is difficult to focus at that point. So, by developing some practical strategies to deal with the controllable factors that affect memory (stress, inattention, planning, etc.), we can get a foothold on the impact of symptoms in your daily life. That is the focus of MAAT."

"Also, we are not going to really know if the memory failure was due to cancer or cancer treatment. So, MAAT will focus solely on how to improve performance in daily life—which we can control."

Ask for the survivor's impressions at this point.

Therapeutic Note: There is a section in the survivor workbook in Visit 1 that reviews different forms of memory and attention (see the heading, "Types of Memory and Attention"). By no means does this provide a complete discussion on the topic; to do so would be too time-consuming. Rather than discussing the basics of cognitive psychology with the survivor, various forms of attention (e.g., sustained, divided) and memory (e.g., verbal auditory, verbal working memory) can be discussed in the context of self-awareness and monitoring of memory problems. All individuals vary in the extent they are more auditory or visual "learners," and this can be reviewed while reviewing the next component of MAAT.

Self-Awareness and Monitoring Memory Problems (Form 1.1)

- The rationale is to increase awareness of "at risk" situations where memory and attention failures can cause problems in daily life.

- Also called "self-monitoring," survivors will keep a brief written record to identify environmental, affective, and cognitive antecedents of memory failures in daily life. This allows for wise selection of MAAT compensatory strategies that will "fit" the survivor's lifestyle. More accurate targeting of memory problems helps improve daily performance on tasks that are valued by the survivor.

- A "memory and attention problem" can be defined as experiencing a perceived lapse remembering a name, placement of an object, steps in a task, etc., or the inability to sustain focus without distraction or to shift focus and return to the task at hand. The survivor should record *"those memory problems or failures that bother you."* Instruct and model form completion. Show the example in the workbook and emphasize simplicity (use only a few words).

Form 1.1 Memory and Attention Problem Record

Memory and Attention Problem Record

Date:_____ Time: _____AM PM

How much did the memory or attention problem bother you?

        0   1   2   3   4   5   6   7   8   9   10

Not at all   Moderately   Extremely

What the memory or attention problem was:

What was happening (where you were, what you were doing, and what the surroundings were like, e.g., noisy, quiet, etc.)

What I felt at the time (Anxious? Tense? Hungry? Tired? Peaceful?)

Memory and Attention Problem Record EXAMPLE

Memory and Attention Problem Record

Date: *11/1/2020*   Time: __*12*__ AM (PM)

How much did the memory and attention problem bother you?

0   1   2   3   4   5   (6)   7   8   9   10

Not at all   Moderately   Extremely

What the memory or attention problem was:

Forgot the PIN to the bankcard I was using, and I also noticed it was a different card.

What was happening (where you were, what you were doing, and what the surroundings were like, e.g., noisy, quiet, etc.)

I was in the city clerk's office, and there was a line with people talking and phones ringing, confusing!

What I felt at the time (Anxious? Tense? Hungry? Tired? Peaceful?)

Felt a little rushed as many people were waiting in line. I was also hungry since I was taking care of a chore on my lunch hour.

- To aid accuracy, the survivor should try to complete the form soon after a failure occurs. If this is not possible, the survivor should try completing forms at the end of the day the failures occur. A copy of the form can be scanned into a mobile device such as a mobile phone or tablet.

- Not every memory and attention failure needs to be recorded. The goal is to get a sample of "at risk" situations; four or five forms will be plenty for discussion time in Visit 2.

Therapeutic Note: Self-awareness is the hallmark of many CBTs so that participants can better identify what factors contribute to the problem they are trying to modify and prevent it from occurring (in this CBT, problems of memory and attention). It is critical to help the survivor understand that identifying external factors that can contribute to memory failures, such as ambient distracting noise, a disorganized environment, and transitioning from home to the workplace, are all environmental factors that can usually be modified. This is important to point out to survivors so they can begin to gain a sense of control. You may find that many survivors undergoing MAAT will forget to bring the workbook if you have an in-office visit with them because they were distracted by something while preparing to leave home. Time of day can also make a difference in memory performance. Glucocorticoids, such as cortisol, play a role in optimal memory performance, and they have a peak release in mid- to late morning.[99] Instruct the survivor to be aware of time-of-day circumstances (it is important to write down the day of the week and time of day on the form), since having many memory failures with critical home or work tasks may be a matter of simply shifting those tasks to times of peak glucocorticoid release (morning hours).

Also, be aware of and discuss with the survivor "internal antecedents" or risk factors for memory failure in daily life such as being tired, hungry, or anxious. It is well known that fatigue contributes to CRCI,[16] but low glucose levels or simply the distraction of hunger can also contribute to memory failures.

One survivor undergoing MAAT noted that she had memory and attention problems in the midafternoon while working online from home, which was where most of her working hours were spent. She found that while she could eat her lunch at any time, she often brought her lunch to her workstation. More often than not, she became distracted with new work tasks on her computer and the hours would speed by without her eating. Upon review of her Memory and Attention Problem Records (Form 1.1), we agreed to make a simple change in the environment: She scheduled lunch for a specific time daily and ate at the dining room table only. This form of stimulus control, or managing the cues in the environment for eating behavior and keeping them separate from the cues for working behavior (the computer workstation), helped to reduce distraction, and she reported better work focus and performance. Feel free to share this and other anecdotes with survivors to stress the importance of self-awareness.

Progressive Muscle Relaxation

- The rationale for PMR is to build the skill of self-regulating autonomic arousal so as to reduce interference with attention. Improved attention leads to improved encoding/learning of information for subsequent recall.

- You can provide the survivor with a digital audio file that you record for daily practice, or you can use any number of PMR recordings available online (explained below).

- Make sure you know well the rationale for PMR in MAAT. These details are not vital to convey to survivors, but you should understand this basic research knowledge and be able to discuss it with survivors who are curious and have questions. For instance, it has long been known that anxiety and stress responding interferes with attention and memory.[100–102] During the stress response, changes in brain activity such as diversion of cerebral blood flow and inhibition of glucose utilization in the hippocampus (a structure critical to memory consolidation) occur.[103] Habitual stress responding may play both an etiologic and maintenance role in CRCI.[104] Moreover, prefrontal neural function and cognitive performance are linked through neurovisceral integration (heart rate variability), which suggests that self-regulation skills training can aid cognitive and behavioral task performance.[105] PMR, when combined with mnemonic strategy training, may enhance memory performance.[106]

- The purpose of PMR is to overlearn the process of letting go of muscle tension in daily life. This involves increasing one's mindfulness of muscle tension in daily activity and "letting go of muscles that are not necessary for the activity at hand." Holding excessive muscle tension can increase sympathetic output of the autonomic nervous system, giving rise to the physiological changes in the brain and body discussed in the prior bullet point. PMR will help the survivor to achieve autonomic balance in daily life (Figure 1.1). PMR is intended to cultivate lower baseline arousal and achieve optimal arousal, not under- or over-arousal. Discuss autonomic balance here. Point out that the sympathetic branch tends to act quickly and stay activated, but it cannot go on indefinitely; the parasympathetic branch will eventually activate to restore energy. Relaxed muscles will activate parasympathetic activity and achieve balance.

- Explain to the survivor that daily PMR practice will help improve awareness of relaxing muscles "all the time, in daily life." During practice with an audio file, one can easily achieve deep relaxation. Emphasis is on daily practice to foster necessary learning through repetition. However, more importantly, repetitive practice allows the survivor to apply skills of relaxing muscles during activity—just like an athlete who relaxes some muscles but tenses others to perform optimally, such as a quarterback throwing a football, a basketball player taking a shot, or a runner who relaxes facial and neck muscles during a sprint but uses leg muscles

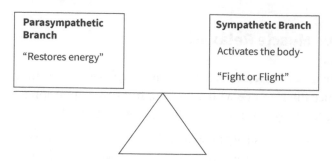

Figure 1.1 Autonomic nervous system: "autopilot"

explosively. Non-athletic examples can include not holding excessive tension in shoulders or legs while working at a computer, not shaking or "bouncing" a leg while in a meeting, or avoiding clenching jaw muscles while reading or listening.

- PMR practice involves flexing and relaxing a series of muscle groups (arms, face, etc.). The purpose for flexing a muscle is that it relaxes more after slight flexion (30%).

- If you want to produce an audio recording with your own voice, a protocol for PMR is given in Appendix 2. Read the script slowly, in a low tone of voice. Be certain that if it is a digital audio file, it can be securely transmitted to the patient without risk to their private identity or health information. An alternative can be any of the PMR exercises found online (there are websites noted in the survivor workbook in visit 1). Be sure to select one you have sampled yourself and experienced it in its entirety, or one you personally use or would have a family member use. One suggestion is www.relaxforawhile.com; it is also on Facebook at www.facebook.com/relaxforawhile.

- The survivor should listen to the audio PMR recording daily. Try to pair the practice session with another daily activity to make it an easy-to-remember habit, such as right after or before lunch or dinner. Survivors can listen to the recording on their computer, smartphone, or tablet or other device. Encourage them to use headphones or earbuds, although this is not necessary. They should allow about 25 minutes for practice in a quiet setting. A relaxation log is given here and in the workbook (Form 1.2) so survivors can track their practice sessions.

- Other tips include:
  - Remind the participant not to flex muscles until they hear the word "now." They then flex at about 30% strength, then "drop" muscle tension *quickly* to exaggerate (over-learn) letting go of muscle tension.
  - If a muscle or painful body part does not allow for comfortable flexing, have the survivor simply not flex that body part and just "focus and relax." The intent is to relax muscles, not induce pain. Be practical.
  - Point out that everyone can experience distracting thoughts and that pushing those thoughts out of one's mind is not helpful. Simply observe the thought, but go on listening to the next step. Even if relaxation is not achieved, the exercise is done. Becoming a good relaxer is like going to the gym—it is through

Form 1.2 Relaxation Practice Log

	0	1	2	3	4	5	6	7	8	9	10	
	Not At All Relaxed				Moderately Relaxed					Very Relaxed		

Date	Relaxation Level Before/After (0 to 10)	Type	Comments
___/___/___	/	❑ PMR ❑ quick	
___/___/___	/	❑ PMR ❑ quick	
___/___/___	/	❑ PMR ❑ quick	
___/___/___	/	❑ PMR ❑ quick	
___/___/___	/	❑ PMR ❑ quick	
___/___/___	/	❑ PMR ❑ quick	
___/___/___	/	❑ PMR ❑ quick	

the accumulation of exercise sessions that strength is built; you don't have to be your strongest at every single weightlifting session. Similarly, relaxation skills are built over the course of many exercise sessions. Encourage the survivor not to feel pressured to be completely relaxed with each practice session.

Therapeutic Note: PMR is an attempt to help survivors gain good self-regulation skills, as the previous bulleted points indicate. Relaxation skills are much more than listening to the PMR audio once per day. The intent is to apply the skill in daily life, essentially by keeping muscles relaxed during daily activity and enhancing mindfulness of how one holds one's muscles. In our experience many survivors will report favoring PMR practice with the audio track over "quick relaxation," the method taught in Visit 2. This is fine; no relaxation method is superior to another. The bottom line of this component of MAAT is to help survivors learn to cultivate lower levels of arousal to enhance focused attention and to minimize stress as a source of interference to attention, encoding, and later recall of material remembered.

Model dialogue:

"The last thing we'll go over today is applied relaxation training, or progressive muscle relaxation. The intent of this strategy is to help you gain a skill for better managing or regulating your body's stress response. As we discussed previously, blood flow changes can occur in the brain that affect regions involved in memory. Have you done any relaxation strategies before?"

Allow time for explanation; inquire what types. Note: Many individuals have some experience with relaxation methods during a demonstration or class, but often they are not instructed in applying it in daily life in a mindful, conscientious manner.

"In progressive muscle relaxation (PMR), you'll do an exercise where you lay flat on a mat, couch, or recliner and slowly flex, and relax, a series of muscle groups. An audio recording will guide you through. The reason for flexing is that muscles relax more after they have been flexed slightly. The intent here is to have you be a good muscle relaxer, not only while listening to the exercise recording but in daily life. When we keep muscles tense, this tends to activate the 'fight or flight' branch of a part of our nervous system."
(Point to the autonomic nervous system in Figure 1.1; you may explain more about the autonomic nervous system—or "auto pilot," to convey its function briefly—if time permits).

"By contrast, relaxing muscles and avoiding excessive tension can restore balance. The idea is not to be so relaxed you are sleepy and unresponsive, but to get the best level of arousal for performance."

Ask for questions, clarifications, or experiences with relaxation effects on memory.

Homework

- The survivor workbook has a Homework Task Sheet (Form 1.3) to help track homework completion. Refer to that with the survivor. The homework assignments are:
  - Review the participant workbook Introduction and Visit 1.
  - Complete Memory and Attention Problem Records (see Form 1.1; four or five of them is plenty).
  - Practice with the PMR audio file daily. Emphasize repetition (rather than perfection) and being mindful and aware of letting go of muscle tension in daily life.
- The workbook has explanations of different types of memory that are not covered in Visit 1 with the clinician due to time constraints. However, you should

be familiar with that content in order to review it with the participant in Visit 2 if questions arise.

- Remember the basic point of the workbook. The readings are intended to review and reinforce the concepts covered. There is much information to cover, and this is with individuals with memory complaints. Keep points simple. Reassure survivors that even if they don't remember important points in the visit, it is all in the workbook, organized visit by visit. The workbook is always available for reference and looking things up.

- Schedule Visit 2.

Form 1.3 Homework Task Sheet

Day: Homework Task	1	2	3	4	5	6	7	8	9	10	11	12	13	14
Assigned reading														
Self-awareness monitoring of memory and attention problems														
Self-Instructional Training														
Progressive muscle relaxation														
Quick relaxation														
Internal verbal rehearsal strategies (SIT, rhymes, spaced rehearsal, etc.) List here:														
External strategies (keeping a schedule, memory routine, pacing, fatigue management, etc.) List here:														

Homework Task Sheet (Example)

Day: Homework Task	1	2	3	4	5	6	7	8	9	10	11	12	13	14
Assigned reading	✓	✓	✓											
Self-awareness monitoring of memory and attention problems	✓	✓	✓	✓	✓	✓	✓							
Self-Instructional Training	✓		✓	✓			✓							
Progressive muscle relaxation														
Quick relaxation														
Internal verbal rehearsal strategies (SIT, rhymes, spaced rehearsal, etc.) List here:														
External strategies (keeping a schedule, memory routine, pacing, fatigue management, etc.) List here:														

Visit 2

Agenda and Clinician Checklist

1. *Review MAAT Reading, Relaxation and Quick Relaxation Review, Rehearsal*
   ___ MAAT reading questions.
   ___ Review PMR practice, ask about mindfulness of tense muscles in daily life.
   ___ Rationale, instruction, and rehearsal of quick relaxation.
2. *Review of Self-Monitoring, Effects of Context, Senses, and Memory Problems*
   ___ Review self-monitoring rationale, reinforce effort to keep records.
   ___ Identify the types of memory or attention failures (e.g., verbal-auditory, visual-attention, recall of written or auditory information, ability to follow instructions).
   ___ Identify environmental factors such as ambient noise, light, or other distractions.
   ___ Identify inner states such as emotions (anxiety, frustration, etc.), fatigue, hunger, pain, nausea.
   ___ Summarize types of memory failures, ask confirmation from survivor.
3. *Internal Strategy: Self-Instructional Training (SIT)*
   ___ Review rationale for compensatory strategies (prevent or reduce impact of the memory/attention failure in daily life).
   ___ Review rationale of SIT, model, rehearse.
   ___ Discuss real-world applications and how to practice in important and less important situations (over-rehearse).
4. *Homework*
   ___ Apply quick relaxation to everyday life—not to avoid anxiety or stress but to confront it with appropriate (not excessive) arousal.
   ___ Apply SIT in everyday tasks, even simple ones, to grow accustomed to the strategy.

Review MAAT Reading, Relaxation and Quick Relaxation Review, Rehearsal

- Review any questions the survivor has from reading over Visit 1 in the MAAT workbook. Take the time to answer questions.

- Review PMR practice, ask how practice went, and verbally reinforce any effort to practice, even if it was not done daily as recommended. Ask about experiences with practice. Ask, *"Which muscles did you notice relaxed the most?"* Inquire if the survivor notices letting go of tension in daily life. *"Are you more mindful or aware of letting muscle tension go in day-to-day activity?"*

- The point is to reinforce the notion that PMR is to increase self-awareness (or mindfulness) of arousal self-regulation in real-world activity, not simply listening to the PMR audio recording. Stressing this is important throughout MAAT.

- If the survivor has not completed PMR practice, simply ask about their awareness or mindfulness of muscle tension in daily life. It may be that they will prefer quick relaxation, which is detailed in this visit.

- This will lead into the explanation and rationale of "quick relaxation," which is a form of cue-controlled relaxation. The intent of quick relaxation is to cultivate a lower and optimal level of arousal throughout the day that is not contingent upon stress or performance demands. That is, it makes little sense to apply relaxation skills only when stressed or over-aroused. Catecholamines (epinephrine and norepinephrine) and other classes of hormones associated with the stress response (e.g., cortisol of the glucocorticoid class) tend to chemically act quickly and sustain their action for longer periods of time. When released in high amounts, catecholamines can interfere with optimal cognitive function, such as hippocampal function associated with verbal recall. Using brief (five seconds to five minutes) relaxation methods throughout the day cultivates a lower level of arousal to begin with, before a stressful trigger is encountered.

- That being said, it is unwise to have extremely low arousal (to the point of being sleepy) since this obviously impairs alertness and sharpness of attention, encoding, processing speed, and recall. This is illustrated in Figure 2.1. This is the well-known "inverted U" arousal-performance curve created by early 20th-century psychologists Yerkes and Dodson, who in 1908 hypothesized that, at least for complex tasks with greater cognitive demand, arousal at optimal levels is desirable to produce peak performance.[107] It is important to distinguish stress from arousal, in that stress is generally considered a mismatch between desired arousal for the performance demand, but this is a discussion beyond our purposes here. Just be sure to emphasize that quick relaxation and PMR are methods to help self-regulate arousal and enhance mindfulness arousal that can help aid cognitive performance.

Model dialogue for introducing quick relaxation may go something like this:

"Here's where we introduce quick or 'cue-controlled' relaxation. This is a relaxation strategy that you apply throughout the day. There is no practice with a recording; it takes just seconds and is intended to help you maintain relaxation, in spite of stress. This will help you apply the muscle relaxation you've been working on and improve your mindfulness of keeping muscles relaxed. You can do this in five seconds, or in five minutes, or longer, if you want to take more time."

(Pause and answer any questions.)

"As you may know, chemicals released into the bloodstream under stress are quick-acting and long-acting—this makes sense if you were trying to get away from danger. However, in everyday 21st-century life, it is not often that we need such alarm reactions. Strong

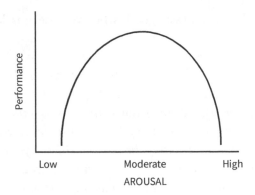

Figure 2.1 Arousal performance curve

stress responses can build up over the course of a day. With quick relaxation, we want you to nearly constantly be mindful of keeping muscles relaxed that you don't need to use and keep a steady, slow pace of breathing. Use the strategy to prevent large buildups of stress reactions, which, as you know, can have a negative effect on memory and attention. In other words, cultivate lower arousal BEFORE stress events come up. Not so that you are sleepy, but maintaining relaxation for focus and 'optimal or best performance.' Here's how you do it."

(Pause and answer any questions. Show the survivor Figure 2.1.)

Quick Relaxation Instructions and Model Dialogue

"Remember, you can do this quick technique in five seconds or five minutes—we'll do about the three- or four-minute version now."

Therapeutic Note: When conducting relaxation techniques in office or videoconference visits, be sure to gradually slow the cadence of your speech and lower the volume and tone of your voice through the exercise. "Slow and low" is the rule of thumb in therapeutic vocal behavior in relaxation induction. Emphasize saying the word "relax" when you see the survivor's chest depress with exhalation in the respiratory cycle. By doing this, you can aid pacing of breathing and associate the word "relax" with the deepest possible state of relaxation—the point at which exhalation is completed, just prior to activating the diaphragm for the next breath.

"Sit in a relaxed position, with your hands comfortably supported in your lap. Remember, you can do this standing up, in line at the bank or grocery store, sitting at a meeting, or riding in a car. You can even be driving a car. Obviously you would not close your eyes for deep relaxation, but you can relax unnecessary muscle tension even in the middle of a serious task like that."

"First, imagine your spine as a freestanding coat rack in a corner—nice and straight. Imagine if we draped a trench coat over the coat rack, it would just flop. Let your muscles flop over your spine—that is, like the coat rack. So, straight spine, loose muscles over this."

(Allow survivor to do this, and say "good" when you see muscle tension leave their shoulders.)

"Next, just close your eyes or stare at a spot straight ahead, and scan your body for any tension, and focus on releasing the tension. Starting at the top of your head . . . Imagine warm relaxing energy or light coming down and going into the muscles of your scalp . . . pushing out the tension . . . relaxing . . . each muscle . . . as it goes . . . smoothing out your forehead, warming . . . relaxing the top and sides of your scalp . . . the back of your head . . . now down into your neck . . . over your temples . . . warming your face like nice warm sunshine . . . now into your jaw . . . allowing it to drop . . . now feel the warm, relaxing energy . . . move into the front of your neck . . . loosening the muscles . . . now warming and flowing through your shoulders . . . pushing out the tension . . . across your upper back . . . across your chest . . . let the muscles become loose . . . warm . . . comfortable . . . and relaxed. Let the relaxation flow . . . into your arms . . . down . . . down . . . warming . . . into your elbows . . . now your forearms . . . down . . . down into your hands . . . warming them . . . pushing the tension out . . . now relaxing . . . each finger . . . so your hands . . . are . . . completely . . . relaxed."

(Pause.)

"Now let the relaxing energy . . . flow down and through your back . . . pushing out the tension as it goes . . . warming, relaxing . . . into your lower back . . . across your chest . . . stomach . . . warming and relaxing your sides . . . letting each muscle go . . . now into your hips . . . pushing out the tension in your upper legs . . . warming . . . relaxing as it goes . . . flowing down, down . . . relaxing . . . each muscle as it goes . . . into your knees . . . now into your lower legs . . . relaxing your calves . . . relaxing . . . warming as it goes . . . now the warm, relaxing energy flows into your feet . . . so now . . . you are completely . . . relaxed.

(Pause.)

"Now . . . just notice your breathing . . . do not change your breathing . . . just notice it . . . allow your breathing to become slower . . . as you exhale . . . imagine you breathe out any remaining tension . . . allow all muscles to relax more . . . and more . . . each time you exhale . . . slowly . . . becoming more . . . and more . . . relaxed. Each time you breathe in . . . you can say to yourself silently . . . 'I am' . . . and as you breathe out, you can say . . . 'relaxed.'"

(Say "relaxed" in a drawn out manner about three times)

"'I am . . . re . . . laxed.' 'I am . . . re . . . laxed' . . . 'I am . . . re . . . laxed' . . . Just continue this for seven or eight more breaths on your own . . . then . . . let me know when you are finished."

(Allow completion. When the survivor opens his or her eyes, ask, *"Which muscles let go of tension?"*)

Point out that the *exhaling* portion of quick relaxation is the most important component with respect to inducing relaxation and "letting go of tension on the fly." Encourage the survivor to use a quick "I am" (on the inhale) and "re . . . laxed" on the exhale procedure several times per hour throughout the day—again, regardless of stressors in the environment. In short, the idea is to cultivate optimal arousal and focus. Emphasis is on simply being aware of muscle tension and relaxing unnecessary tension.

Review of Self-Monitoring, Effects of Context, Senses, and Memory Problems

Therapeutic Note: The point of self-monitoring is simple: to help identify antecedent conditions under which memory and attention problems interfere with functioning. Reiterate this when going over the self-monitoring samples.

Look for patterns of what times memory and attention failures occur and what sensory modalities are affected. For example, if the survivor reports problems of not remembering conversations or details in a meeting, then verbal-auditory encoding and recall may be a problem. If they have difficulty following the steps of written instructions, then recall of written material or working memory for sequential tasks (steps) may be a problem. Alternatively, visual-spatial memory problems can lead to problems of getting lost or difficulty following a sequence of visual cues (e.g., missing a turn or exit while driving). Examine if auditory or visual distractions pose a challenge for the survivor, or if he or she "gets lost" in a set of steps in a task such as cooking. Do they experience processing speed problems such that they can't keep up with conversations at meetings or while socializing? Look for times of day—are the problems typically occurring before meals, when the survivor is hungry and blood glucose levels are low? Are they occurring late in the day, when the survivor is tired? Note the various types of difficulties under various conditions, and engage the survivor in identifying "at risk" conditions. This is a critical step to help survivors identify just where cognitive failures are likely to occur so they can pick the compensatory strategies that work best for their unique pattern of cognitive difficulty.

- Review the rationale, as stated in the prior paragraphs, and offer verbal praise for any effort in completing the self-monitoring and self-awareness exercise. If it wasn't completed, or if the survivor left the forms at home, ask if they recall any failures, and use the line of inquiry outlined in the rest of this bulleted list. While not ideal, it at least begins the process of raising self-awareness and mindfulness of the conditions under which cognitive problems may arise.

- Identify types of memory failures (e.g., verbal-auditory, visual attention, recall of written information, ability to follow written or oral instruction). What sensory modality—visual, auditory, even olfactory—does the survivor tend to use in memory?

- Identify environmental factors such as ambient noise, light, or other distractions. For example, if reading in dim lighting, perhaps simple visual acuity interfered with encoding, or maybe the noise in the environment is too much.

- Identify inner states, such as anxiety, frustration, hunger, fatigue, or pain. Did these states contribute to poor attention and distraction and interfere with encoding or recall?

- As usual, summarize possible contributors and ask the survivor if these hypotheses are plausible: *"So it seems that you have more memory problems during midday, just after lunch, when you may feel tired after eating and many people are busy in your office area. Most of the problems are remembering steps in the tasks you have to do at your desk. Could it be that auditory distraction is affecting your focused attention? Is this something you experience?"*

Internal Strategy: Self-Instructional Training (SIT)

Therapeutic Note: Compensatory strategies are introduced in this visit. "Compensatory" means they are intended not to restore memory function but to help individuals *compensate* for cognitive dysfunction that can lead to negative consequences in daily life. This was explained in Visit 1 and is reiterated here. Throughout MAAT, the basic format of compensatory strategy presentation is to review the rationale, demonstrate real-world use through modeling, and rehearse or review with the survivor how they will apply the strategy in daily life. This is detailed here with the first compensatory strategy, Self-Instructional Training (SIT). As stated earlier, the following instructions are guidelines, and not all content needs to be covered if time does not permit. Keep your instructions simple and to the point, and have open discussion with the survivor to optimize learning.

- Self-Instructional Training (SIT) is a form of "covert modeling" that refers to verbalizing the mental steps or "internal dialogue" involved in carrying out a task. The intent of this compensatory strategy in MAAT is to help participants improve their ability to maintain sustained attention. Improving sustained attention can enhance awareness and reduce distraction that can interfere with task completion or encode reading content. In short, SIT involves "talking through" a task to prevent cognitive distraction from impairing task performance and to aid in later recall of task steps. In addition to enhancing sustained attention, SIT can potentially enhance attention shift from one focus to another and thus aid in performance of complex tasks.

- SIT was originally designed and used successfully to help impulsive children maintain self-control.[108] Other applications include enhancement of sustained attention among test-anxious college students,[109] older adults with problem-solving deficits,[110] young children with reading comprehension deficits,[111,112] and at least one adult with attention deficits following brain injury.[113] While most of these studies are somewhat dated, the theoretical and practical tenets of SIT make it highly applicable to the problem of CRCI.

- Teaching SIT consists of several discrete steps. The clinician first models the procedure, and then the survivor rehearses it and they discuss how SIT will be used in daily life. Steps are outlined here.

Step 1: Explaining the Rationale

In this step the clinician explains the basis for why SIT can help maintain focused attention:

"Self-Instructional Training, or 'self-talk,' is basically this: talking to yourself as you do things. It is like being your own sports play-by-play announcer. It sounds funny, but research suggests it improves attention if we learn to talk ourselves through tasks. Older people with memory problems have benefited from this as well as children with attention and impulse control problems—they tend to stay on task better with self-instruction. Have you heard of it? Most of us have occasionally talked to ourselves out loud to get a task done."

(Survivors may say they have done this naturally—allow some time to explain.)

"Here's how Self-Instructional Training or 'talking to yourself' works. The brain has a set of 'executive functions' that help us control and manage behavior. This helps us complete goal-directed behavior such as getting dressed, preparing and cooking a meal, or packing a lunch. 'Self-instruction' is an 'inner voice' that helps us in carrying out tasks with many steps and stay on task so it can get completed. Many people who have undergone cancer treatment find they may have difficulty focusing on the steps in a task and may skip one or get distracted and not remember which step they were on. Self-Instructional Training will help to make that 'inner voice' more noticeable and help you improve your awareness and task focus."

(The clinician should ask for an example from self-monitoring, if applicable.)

"Another reason for Self-Instructional Training is to reduce the effects of negative or unhelpful thinking at the first sign of distraction, thing like 'Here I go again; my attention is horrible!' Therefore, the procedure you will learn now will help you use 'self-talk' to stay focused."

(Answer any questions.)

Step 2: Modeling and Rehearsal

"We will practice this. I will show you what I say to myself as I do a task (cognitive modeling), then you will do the task after if you like."

(Using SIT, demonstrate filling out Form 2.1. Speak out loud, describing to yourself what you are doing.)

"Alright, what is it I have to do? I'm going to fill out this form. Okay, let me see . . . first I will fill in my name . . . Robert, R-O-B-E-R-T . . . Good. Now my date of birth. Good. Make sure I have the right year . . . yes, I do. Now I move down to my address. OK, my address is 15 Oak Drive. Whoops, I put 20! That's OK, I will just erase it and fix it to 15."

Form 2.1 Practice Form for Self-Instructional Training Demonstration

Today's Date_____

Name_____   Date of Birth_____
Address

_____

_____

_____

_____

Phone Numbers
Home_____   Mobile_____
Work_____

- Some survivors will decline practicing this in the office with the model form, and it is alright if they don't. SIT is a simple technique, but strongly emphasize that it should be used often so it becomes a routine or habit. SIT can be carried out with any number of practice tasks, such as copying a list, reconciling a checking account balance, cooking, doing important tasks at work that require sequential steps, or solving math problems of everyday life. The practice will be its application in everyday life.

- Note that in the dialogue you are essentially a play-by-play announcer of the internal cognitive experience of task completion. Model falling off task so that you can emphasize positive self-talk such as *"I'm distracted by noise, but that's OK, I'm refocusing now . . . let's fill out the address section."* This is an important aspect of SIT. Rather than modeling negative self-talk that reinforces anxiety about attention and memory problems (e.g., *"I always forget the ZIP code! This is so embarrassing. I'll never have the mind I had before chemotherapy!"*), focus on matter-of-factly and gently guiding attention back to the task at hand (e.g., *"That's OK, I'll just correct this. Yes, now I'll put in the ZIP code."*).

- Repetition is believed to be an important factor in developing the compensatory skill of SIT. Homework practice for SIT should be practical because it is intended for use in daily life. Ask the survivor which tasks they will use this for that will be meaningful to them. Ask how they will actually use it.

- Encourage survivors to "talk to themselves" during most daily tasks. Use the phrase *"Practice with the mundane, as well as the meaningful."* That is, use SIT in virtually all tasks such as tying shoes, getting keys out of one's pocket to unlock a door, sorting and folding laundry, cleaning and organizing clutter, or entering phone numbers. Remind survivors that daily tasks that may seem trivial can be opportunities to hone their SIT skills. In this way, SIT will become automatic and in better form when the pressure is on to perform well in important, non-trivial tasks. We have found that this makes an impression with most survivors and SIT becomes a new habit.

Homework

- Practice quick relaxation in everyday life—not in a reactive way but to cultivate optimal arousal *before* stressful circumstances arise and to optimize attention and concentration.

- Apply SIT in everyday tasks, even simple ones, to grow accustomed to the strategy.

- Remember the basic point of the workbook. The readings are intended to review and reinforce concepts covered in the visit, and all material in the Visit 2 reading will be review.

Visit 3

Agenda and Clinician Checklist

1. *Quick Relaxation Review*
___ Ask about mindfulness and ability to relax muscles in everyday activity.
2. *Review Application of Self-Instructional Training (SIT)*
___ Review use of SIT in real-world situations; review examples of use.
___ If not used or rehearsed, identify reasons why, barriers, and modifications.
3. *Internal Strategy: Verbal Rehearsal Strategies (Verbal Rehearsal, Spaced Rehearsal, Chunking, and Rhymes)*
___ Rationale: rehearsal, spaced rehearsal, and other methods.
___ Identify examples in survivor's daily life; rehearse.
4. *Cognitive Restructuring: Realistic Probabilities and Decatastrophizing*
___ Rationale: Emotions are the product of cognitive appraisal, thought.
___ Identifying and challenging styles of thinking that maintain distress can aid emotional coping, not make the world perfect.
___ Review probability estimation.
___ Review decatastrophizing.
5. *Homework*
___ Apply chosen compensatory strategy or combination.
___ Use and evaluate probability estimation, decatastrophizing in daily life.

Quick Relaxation Review

- Ask about experiences with applying quick relaxation. Inquire about mindfulness or awareness of muscle tension in daily life, and if they were able to let go of excessive tension, or at least attempt it (e.g., *"What muscles were you able to relax in daily activity? Are you more aware of how you hold your body?"*). Remember to reinforce the effort, not so much if quick relaxation "worked" or not. You may also ask how close they came to achieve feelings similar to the progressive muscle relaxation (PMR) audio recording—were they able to "mimic" feelings associated with deep relaxation? Remember also that quick relaxation is to cultivate optimal levels of arousal for better self-regulation. It is not intended as a method to use only after one gets stressed.

- Emphasis is placed on practice and process, working toward the goal of mindfulness of carrying tension, and letting it go. No one is expected to perfect this skill. It is sometimes useful to ask if the survivor has observed others in daily life holding muscle tension or fidgeting with anxiety. Ask if this helps increase awareness of their own tension-holding behavior (reverse modeling). Problem-solve as necessary.

Review Application of Self-Instructional Training (SIT)

- Inquire how the participant applied SIT and in what situations. Did it help with staying on task, or at least coming back to task after "drifting"? Was it applied in any of the situations reviewed in self-awareness monitoring? Allow the survivor to discuss their experiences and reinforce effort for applying the strategy. Problem-solve and modify as needed. If it wasn't useful, emphasize there are other compensatory strategies that can help with coping and there may be other applications of SIT in the future.

Internal Strategy: Verbal Rehearsal Strategies (Verbal Rehearsal, Spaced Rehearsal, Chunking, and Rhymes)

- Verbal rehearsal consists of both overt rehearsal (repeating out loud) and covert rehearsal (repeating to oneself silently) to aid with retention and recall of auditory and written information. In short, it is a method of repeated rehearsal to commit important information to short-term memory long enough so that some action can be carried out—for example, rehearsing a telephone number or street address until one can either call the number or write it down, or to help consolidate the association between a name and a face. An interesting case of using verbal rehearsal was with a participant in early MAAT research. This particular breast cancer survivor worked as a dental hygienist who wore standard safety equipment of gloves, mask, and safety glasses and thus could not conveniently remove these items to write down information during a busy day with numerous patients (not to mention that her hands were in people's mouths much of the work day). With some frequency, staff might interrupt her to ask a question or to carry out a task when she had a moment. Spaced rehearsal, detailed later in the chapter, became a convenient method to help her meet job responsibilities.

- You don't need to rehearse each of these methods with the survivor in the office. Do cover spaced rehearsal and practice with the mastery experience seen later in the chapter (memorizing the clinic office number), but reviewing the others briefly in the office and reviewing the survivor workbook at home should suffice. It is better for the survivor to feel confident with one method rather than unconfident and shaky with many.

- Verbal rehearsal methods used in MAAT consist of (1) simple overt or covert rehearsal and repetition; (2) spaced rehearsal (repeating information with successively longer time intervals between repetitions); (3) chunking (grouping auditory or written bits of information); and (4) using rhymes to deepen encoding with emotions such as humor.

- The rationale for verbal rehearsal may go as follows:

"Many people find that after cancer treatment they may have difficulty recalling small facts such as names of people they recently met, phone numbers, or other auditory or written information. Part of the problem may be attending to the information long enough so that it can be stored in memory to recall later. A way to help this storage process involves repeating the information out loud or silently until the information can either be written down or you take some action with it. For example, when meeting someone, you repeat their name before you state yours. Another example is repeating a phone number out loud once you have heard it so that you can call the number, or write it down."

Verbal Rehearsal: Overt and Covert Rehearsal

- Instruction in verbal rehearsal comprises two steps: the clinician (1) explains what to do, and then (2) models the behavior. Short, concise explanations are best, and generally the more rehearsal the participant has, the better. Remember, refer to the participant workbook where these methods are detailed. Model dialogue is as follows:

"Let's practice verbal and silent rehearsal of new information. I will show you some ways to do this. Then, you will try it, and we will rehearse it until it becomes automatic for you."

"First, we will use an example of being introduced to someone, or if someone introduces themselves. When someone states his or her name, you can repeat it either with a greeting or as a question as if to politely clarify that you heard the name correctly. For example, if someone says, 'Hello, I'm Jane Jackson,' you can say, 'Hello, Jane Jackson, I'm (name).' Or, you could respond, 'Jane Jackson? Hi, I'm (name).' It's important that as you say this you look the other person in the eye so a name–face association has a chance to form."

- The clinician should model cordial, assertive behavior. The point is to promote the use of verbal rehearsal—repeating a name in this case—in a manner to minimize social awkwardness. Emphasis is placed on smiling, a forward lean without getting too close to the other party, and using an assertive (vs. passive or aggressive) tone. The clinician should touch on these points but not lose the main point, which is to *repeat the name so that it can be held in attention long enough to be stored for later recall.*

Spaced Rehearsal and Chunking

- "Spaced rehearsal" simply refers to making the time interval slightly longer between each repetition—that is, "spacing" the intervals longer and longer between repetitions of the thing to be learned and recalled later. This method aids encoding through the mental "exercise" of "testing" recall. The example in the MAAT workbook illustrates this with remembering a name: "When you hear it, you repeat to yourself, 'Alice Jones,' and then you wait three seconds and repeat, 'Alice Jones.' Then wait seven seconds and repeat, 'Alice Jones,' then again with an even longer interval. Visually, this would appear something like this: "Alice Jones" . . . "Alice Jones" . . . . . "Alice Jones" . . . . "Alice Jones" . . . . "Alice Jones" . . . . "Alice Jones." This can be used along with chunking as seen later in the chapter.

- Short-term learning and recall of complex numbers can be aided by "chunking" numbers. For example, the phone number 333-364-7641 can be repeated as "333 . . . 364 . . . 76 . . . 41." In other words, individual numbers are "chunked" into larger numbers (e.g., four digits, "7641," becomes two numbers, "76" and "41," or 000 becomes "triple zero"). Radio and TV ads do this to increase the chances listeners will remember the number. The clinician should explain this to the participant and rehearse.

Therapeutic Note: We have found in MAAT that using our office or clinic phone number for in-office practice of spaced rehearsal allows for a mastery experience for survivors. It is useful information if the survivor needs to call to reschedule an appointment. Have the participant rehearse spaced rehearsal until they have mastered the office number and are confident. "Quiz" them a minute or two later by asking for the number, then ask again later once or twice in the visit and at the end of the visit. This builds confidence in using spaced rehearsal. Also, in current times of mobile devices, it is easy to not bother to memorize phone numbers because of electronic lists of contact names—simply tap on the call icon or use a voice command and the call is under way. Have the survivor practice spaced rehearsal at home by committing to memory two important phone numbers (family or friends) as homework.

Rhymes

- For centuries, nursery rhymes have capitalized on phonetic associations to enhance encoding and recall: "One, two, buckle my shoe . . . three, four, shut the door." Therefore, in MAAT, rhymes are used to remember names, numbers, or tasks.

- **Rhyming names.** This is simple with simple names, such as, "Jane from Maine," "Dan fan," "Doug on rug," etc. However, it may be a bit trickier with longer or unusual names. Encourage creativity, even rhymes that may even be unflattering to the person whose name you are trying to remember. Emotion deepens memory.

Adding an emotional element to the name–person association, such as humor, can deepen encoding—for example, "Maureen the queen," "Bryant the tyrant," or "Denise has geese." Some of these rhymes may imply the opposite of personal character or be simple nonsense, "Josh squash" or "Marquee on a lark-ie."

- **Rhyming tasks.** A cancer survivor in previous MAAT research indicated she had difficulty remembering the medications in her morning routine. This was critical as she also had diabetes and needed to balance several medications to minimize complications. She came up with a rhyme that was silly but meaningful to her: "To be like Edison, take your medicine." She repeated this several times each night before going to bed as she prepared her pills for the next day. On awakening, it was nearly the first thing she repeated, if not the first. This commonsense verbal routine resulted in greater medication adherence.

- **Musical rhymes with melodies.** Again, this is simple and has been used in education for centuries to enhance memory—the alphabet song, for example. Think of the power of advertising jingles coming out of Madison Avenue for McDonald's, Coca-Cola, or automobiles. Emphasize simplicity and using either familiar or improvised melodies to combine with rhymes, spaced rehearsal, chunking, etc.

Cognitive Restructuring: Realistic Probabilities and Decatastrophizing

Therapeutic Note: Cognitive restructuring (CR) refers to the therapeutic strategy of identifying, challenging, and modifying maladaptive thoughts, appraisals, assumptions, beliefs, or attitudes that can maintain emotional distress. It is at the heart of most cognitive-behavioral therapies (CBTs) and involves a collection of techniques ranging from simple education to guided inquiry through Socratic questioning. At some level, all emotional reactions are produced by rapid appraisals and evaluations of the outside world, which leads to emotional responding so that appropriate, adaptive action can take place. However, at times, misconception, appraisal errors, misattributions, or negatively biased "thinking habits" can lead to maladaptive emotions and actions. Thus, the common goals of all CR methods are to lead survivors or others to:

- Make distinctions between thoughts and feelings. Too often, at least in English-speaking Western culture, the words "think" and "feel" are used synonymously: "I *feel* my memory is declining ever since chemotherapy." This is a thought, not a feeling.

- Enhance self-awareness of how thoughts influence feelings and how this may lead to unhelpful behaviors, such as giving up when persistence will likely lead to success, or not persisting when a change in goals would be more productive and successful.

- Develop the skill to critically evaluate one's own thinking, beliefs, or assumptions, and change these "on the fly," in the real world, to aid emotional coping and successful adaptation to circumstances.

Contrary to many misunderstandings of CR, it is not a simple matter of the "power of positive thinking." Rather, the intent is to identity rational thought that can improve adaptation to, and optimal coping with, sometimes grave circumstances. In Visit 1, you have already engaged in an important CR method that was intended to have survivors view their cognitive failures in a less catastrophic manner—to at least consider that possibility that not all cognitive failures are caused by CRCI, but many cognitive failures may be caused by more controllable factors such as choice of stress responding, poor organization, or distracting environments. That was the intent of the educational material covered, and comparisons of Table 1.2 and Table 1.3. It is hoped that survivors will begin to more openly challenge misattributions of cognitive failures to chemotherapy alone and reduce selective focus on memory failures that confirm catastrophic beliefs.

For clinicians well versed in CBT, this section will serve as a review. For those inexperienced in using CR, seeking supervision and instruction from an experienced psychologist colleague or other licensed professional is advised. Reading the references on CBT cited in the introduction is strongly advised. Too often, inexperienced clinicians launch into CR expecting patients to have rapid belief or attitude change. The result may involve getting caught in stalemates or arguing, which will only entrench maladaptive assumptions, beliefs, or attitudes. In MAAT, CR is introduced to the survivor through the review of two simple methods of CR or "thought challenges:" "probability estimation" and "decatastrophizing."

- The rationale for CR is presented as a method to identify and modify thoughts, assumptions, attitudes, or beliefs that may maintain excessive emotional distress and serve as a barrier to optimal emotional coping or resilience. The clinician should be familiar with the written exercises and presentation of materials in the survivor workbook. However, it is not necessary to review this in detail with the survivor in the visit. It is important to, whenever practical, discuss CR to help enhance coping with cognitive problems.

    "We now move on to another strategy—the 'cognitive' part of cognitive–behavioral therapy. In this segment, we will work on methods to help challenge thinking styles or habits that can maintain negative emotion or delay coping with difficult situations: 'cognitive restructuring' or 'thought challenging.' Have you heard of this before?"

- Await the survivor's response. Evaluate their knowledge level. Fit the following explanations to meet their familiarity with CR. You can review with them the "thud in the next room" explanation (in the CR section of Visit 3 of the survivor workbook—you should be familiar with that example) to help illustrate how rapid perceptions, assumptions, and automatic thoughts produce emotional responses.

"We'll work on 2 simple strategies: one is to challenge a natural, human tendency to overestimate the probability something bad could happen with memory failure; the other is 'decatastrophizing.' Are these familiar terms?"

- Await the survivor's response and discuss as appropriate to segue into probability estimation.

Probability Estimation

Probability estimation is a method to identify the real or rational probability a negative event may occur versus the irrational overestimation that some negative event will occur. In general, it makes adaptive sense from a behavioral evolutionary standpoint that human beings naturally tend to overestimate the probability of negative life events. This leads us to be ready for any number of scenarios. Emergency preparedness for disasters and studying for exams are common adaptive examples. However, it becomes maladaptive if the individual over-prepares to the point of exhaustion of resources needed to perform (e.g., "pulls an all-nighter") or avoids situations such as air travel due to possible, but highly improbable, outcomes (e.g., dying in a plane crash). In short, survivors are encouraged to make distinctions between (1) real probabilities or negative consequences of cognitive errors and (2) feared, irrational overestimations of negative consequences.

For example, a survivor may estimate that if they forget to pay a bill on time, their credit rating will be forever scarred and this will result in certain bankruptcy. However, you can ask, *"Out of the last X times you've been late with a bill, how many times did it result in bankruptcy?"* In other words, using simple arithmetic, one can estimate rough probabilities by asking "Out of the last 10 times this has happened, how many times did it result in . . .?"

It is common to overestimate catastrophic outcomes with many things, such as shark attacks or dying in a plane crash. It is not uncommon to ask a room full of adults what the probability is of dying in a plane crash and to hear, "It's low, maybe 1%." However, according to the U.S. Federal Aviation Administration in 2020, there are nearly 44,000 commercial aviation flights per day in the 5.3 million miles of U.S. air space daily (faa.gov). At a 1% rate of probability, that would mean 440 aviation crashes daily. In actual fact, the chance of dying in the next commercial flight one chooses to take is about 1 in 90 million—regardless of how many times one flies (or flying every day for the next 250,000 years before an accident occurs). This is according to Dr. Arnold Barnett, a professor at Massachusetts Institute of Technology who studies air traffic operations and who at one time had a fear of flying (see: https://www.thedailybeast.com/the-great-plane-crash-myth). Of course, it is permissible for us to be nervous or anxious, but it is vital to acknowledge that despite our emotions, the mathematical facts remain the same. You can use these points to illustrate the use of "real probability" estimation in both memory-related and non–memory-related worries.

With respect to memory failures, it may be most helpful to have the survivor learn and practice probability estimation to challenge their *overestimation* that a disastrous consequence may occur due to a memory failure (e.g., "My child's coach will think I am negligent if I forget to pick up my son at practice," "My business will fail because I am doing less for it and others have to take on more duties because of my memory problems").

Decatastrophizing

Decatastrophizing is a method of cognitive coping that is essentially acceptance. In short, while the previous section deals with worries about what *might* happen and the *chances of it happening*, decatastrophizing is a method confronting the most-feared outcome. It is essentially a cognitive process of acknowledging that bad things, regardless of how remote or probable, can and do occur. It is also a fact that despite bad things happening, we somehow go on. Time and the universe continue despite us, with us, or without us. In this sense, decatastrophizing is a method of acknowledging and accepting these facts and helps lessen the emotional burden of always trying to avoid these realities. Catastrophic thinking may theoretically maintain emotional distress or anxiety because the catastrophizer never "finishes the thought." That is, when one thinks of a catastrophic personal outcome due to a memory failure (e.g., "I'll get fired if I forget another meeting, my boss told me!"), the aversive and painful emotional experience associated with that thought may lead the person to cognitively avoid or distract. This reduces painful emotion, but only temporarily. Soon after, the catastrophic thought returns and the cycle repeats.

By contrast, decatastrophizing is a method of eliminating the avoidance and "completing the thought" through confrontation. It is a form of cognitive exposure therapy that numerous studies have shown is the best way to improve anxiety management of worry in the long term.

- To decatastrophize, the simple method is to ask, "Well, what would I do if X were to happen? (answer . . .) Then what would I do? (answer . . .) Then what? (answer . . .) And then what?" In other words, have the survivor ask themselves what they would do if the negative event were to occur. For example, if the memory failure resulted in missing an important work meeting, what would they *actually* do? Repeat "then what?" several times, followed by the next step. You will soon see this places an emphasis on that fact that as time passes, they will likely take steps to mitigate or remedy the consequences of missing the meeting. In short, have them "finish the thought," as explained earlier.

We often take steps to cope with loss or change so that we eventually learn to live with it—we may never get over it, but over time we do learn to live with it. An example of this is the death of a loved one. Death is an unavoidable fact of life, and when our loved ones die we are hurt. We may never be "over" the loss, but eventually, we somehow incorporate, process, and live with their loss and the emotions of no longer having them with us in life. This theme is beyond what may be used in MAAT, but it does illustrate how decatastrophizing can aid emotional coping.

Here is an illustration of the clinician using decatastrophizing. Note how little the clinician has to say:

SURVIVOR: "My memory is so bad I might miss the mandatory staff meeting!"
And then what?
"I would get fired—my boss said so if I miss anymore!"
And after getting fired, what then?
"I would be upset, fall apart!"
And then what?
"Well, I guess I would pack my things, leave the office."
And then what, after you pack, leave?
"I guess I would tell my family and they'd support me."
And then what?
"I'd begin looking for a different job—in fact, I have good ties with another company and they have liked my work. I might call them about past offers."
And then?
"Well, I've learned my happiness is important, my friend has pointed out more flexible hours are good, and I might even like that."
And then what?
"Well, I may get another job. You know, really, the likelihood I would get fired anyway is pretty small—even if I did upset my boss, I've been there a long time and perform well and have more experience than others."

- As seen in this dialogue, frequently after a decatastrophizing sequence, survivors conclude that despite the possibility of a "catastrophic outcome" of a memory failure, the risk of such an outcome may be remote. In addition, the "catastrophe" is lower in magnitude after such an analysis, or if not, there is a strong likelihood of coping after difficulty.

Homework

- Identify which verbal rehearsal compensatory strategies are to be used (or combination) and in what situations. Again, the intent is not to overwhelm the survivor—select *the most practical verbal rehearsal strategy* that fits the survivor's daily demands and preferences.

- Ask the survivor how they might apply probability estimation or decatastrophizing methods to aid in coping with memory problems and daily demands. They are welcome to try the written exercises in Appendix 2 in the workbook, which can be an effective method to enhance learning to challenge automatic thoughts. However, this is not necessary.

- Read and review Visit 3 in the survivor workbook. Feel free to read ahead.

Visit 4

Agenda and Clinician Checklist

1. *Review of Verbal Rehearsal Strategies*
   ___ Ask about what verbal rehearsal strategies were used, for what, when, where.
   ___ Modify as needed.
2. *Review Realistic Probabilities and Decatastrophizing*
   ___ Inquire if these methods helped "rethink" memory problems or barriers.
   ___ Which method appeared to aid coping? How?
3. *External Strategy: Keeping a Schedule and Memory Routines*
   ___ Rationale for keeping a schedule, day planner.
   ___ Keep only one schedule organizer, day views, use pencil (if not electronic), simplify.
   ___ Rationale for keeping memory routines; keep it simple.
   ___ Combining these (routine to *look* at schedule or day planner *daily* to add/change tasks).
4. *Homework*
   ___ Apply chosen compensatory strategy or combination.
   ___ Ask about when and where strategies will be used.

Review of Verbal Rehearsal Strategies

- Review which types of verbal rehearsal methods were applied and with which valued activities. Ask the survivor to detail their use of methods, and be sure to reinforce any attempted use and practical modifications. Allow enough time to review and assess the survivor's perceived usefulness of the strategy.

- Inquire about any modifications of methods that may be necessary. In addition, review whether quick relaxation or just being mindful of tension and arousal regulation aids with attention and memory function or using compensatory strategies.

Review Realistic Probabilities and Decatastrophizing

- In addition to the prior points, review whether identifying and modifying distress-related thoughts has had any positive impact on emotional coping with memory and attention problems. How aware is the survivor of overestimating the likelihood of a negative consequence of a memory failure or inattentive episode? Was the survivor able to catch catastrophic thinking? Ask for specific examples of how it was applied to memory failures, such as, *"Tell me about your experience—did catching your overestimating or catastrophizing change your feelings around memory problems?"* Emphasize that practice will lead to a more natural thought challenge process. Encourage real-world application for real circumstances. If methods were not used, encourage their use or review as necessary to aid in the survivor's understanding of cognitive restructuring.

External Strategy: Keeping a Schedule and Memory Routines

"External strategy" refers to compensatory methods that make use of devices, environmental cues, or reminders to aid memory to perform well at a desired task. These occur external to survivors and may not have a direct impact on cognitive function but will help them to compensate for daily memory problems.

Keeping a Schedule

Keeping a schedule is the first method introduced. In our experience, many individuals bothered by CRCI functioned well in their pre-cancer life, seemingly putting little effort into organizing their time or schedules. Perhaps they did not even use an organized or detailed calendar or day planner. If they did use one, it may have been loosely organized, it may have lacked pertinent detail, or it was inconsistently used (e.g., the survivor didn't carry it with them every day). However, following active cancer treatment and when returning to pre-disease levels of responsibility at home or on the job, omissions of important tasks may occur more frequently. Others may express disappointment in the survivor or even accuse him or her of being negligent or careless with responsibilities. Having a neatly organized schedule suddenly becomes a necessity.

Where to begin? Here are basic points to cover with survivors who may be unfamiliar with using a day planner. Of course, some survivors use a schedule on their mobile phone, tablet, or laptop or keep a neatly organized paper document. If that is the case, simply review some of the following tips to see if they would like to incorporate them. If not, move on with the rest of MAAT. It does not matter if the planner is electronic or paper; the principles of clarity and simplicity remain the same. This section will contain only minimal model dialogue for clinicians; rather, written guidelines on schedule making are listed. These guidelines are also detailed in the participant workbook.

The rationale for keeping a schedule (day planner or electronic calendar application) is to assist survivors in organizing their days so they are not overwhelmed by multiple tasks and so they can develop a regular routine to the greatest extent possible. This is to "remove the burden of having to memorize important tasks and achieve peace of mind these tasks are in the day planner."

1) **Consider using a paper day planner.** Electronic devices such as smartphones, smartwatches, and tablets combine communications technologies and offer a vast array of schedule-making options. However, consider the advantages of an old-fashioned day planner:
   a. It does not have to be charged and will never run out of battery power.
   b. It requires no set-up or software updates.
   c. There is no monthly fee, data charges, or need for Wi-Fi access.

Given these upsides, it is not surprising that many individuals, of all ages, prefer to use a paper day planner. Recommend a format that has *one page for one day*. Avoid day planners with week or month displays because the spaces are not big enough to write in daily tasks or appointments. Conversely, hourly slots allow easy entry of tasks. Most schedules or day planners list all daytime hours on one page, with some space devoted to evening hours:

April 5, 2021

6:00 a.m._____

7:00 a.m._____

8:00 a.m._____

9:00 a.m._____

10:00 a.m._____

11:00 a.m._____

Noon_____

1:00 p.m._____

2:00 p.m._____

3:00 p.m._____

4:00 p.m._____

5:00 p.m._____

6:00 p.m._____

7:00 p.m._____

Evening _____

Of course, survivors will vary in preferences, so any similar format will likely be helpful.

2) **If using a paper schedule, write all entries in** *pencil.* Why? Schedules change. Changes should be expected. Writing in pencil with a good eraser (emphasis here!) allows changes to be made quickly, easily, and neatly so the schedule stays readable. *Keep a pencil with a good eraser in the day planner.* These are all moot points with electronic devices, which are advancing rapidly in terms of simplicity of use.

3) **Keep** *one* **schedule.** The schedule of daily events should be kept in one source, whether paper or electronic. Having two or more schedules leads to confusion because conflicting events could be entered. Keep a schedule for *the whole day*, not just the workday. Evening activities should be scheduled; for example, "5:45 p.m., pick up milk." The schedule should be *kept on one's person at all times.*

   Obviously, some employment requires a worksite schedule, such as health care professionals who must use the electronic health record administered by support staff (this is the lead author's reality). In this case, the personal schedule simply blocks off that time as "work" or the assumption is made that these times are work hours.

4) **Eliminate "to-do" lists.** More often than not, to-do lists never get completed because they don't allow for a visual overview of how much can actually be carried out in a limited time span. Instead, our intent here is to actually schedule when each task is to be done. This will actually force the scheduler to better manage time by prioritizing tasks and realistically budgeting limited time.

5) **Prioritize.** One problem with schedule making that contributes to memory problems is scheduling too many daily tasks in addition to routine tasks. Only the most important new tasks should be added to the schedule.

6) **Schedule routine events first.** Block off meal times, bed times, etc., to ensure established routines. This should be done first. Why? Routines in part reduce "memory burden," and having regular bed and wake times aids circadian rhythm and sleep quality—an important if not critical element in cognitive health.[114] Then, put in "special" daily events for the upcoming time period (week, month, two months, etc.—whatever is realistic and convenient).

7) **Schedule the week.** Set aside weekend or other non-work daytime to schedule the upcoming week. This does not have to be every activity of every day, just the highlights and important things. Do this at the same time each week (such as Sunday at 5 p.m.) to ensure it will be done and not forgotten.

8) *Use* **the schedule.** Help the survivor establish a routine of looking at the schedule daily, such as before or after breakfast or at some starting point of the day. This is based on the principle that it's easier to establish a new habit when it is paired with or placed temporally next to an already established routine. One participant in early MAAT research placed her planner in her bathroom on a

shelf each night before she went to bed. In this way, she could not avoid looking at her schedule when she was done with her morning routine.

9) **Simplify.** Keep the schedule simple. Avoid the temptation to schedule too many tasks. Review the schedule with the survivor and encourage them to schedule only the tasks that are most important and that are most likely to get done.

Memory Routines

Memory routines are behavioral rituals used to reduce the risk of losing objects or to cue critical steps in task performance. Examples of memory routines are:

Placing car or house keys on the same hook *every time* you walk in the door
Placing your purse to the right of the chair leg when you sit down
Keeping your day planner or electronic device in the same spot every bedtime (such as the bathroom example we just mentioned)
Having a routine for locking up your office or shop (e.g., shut off computers; check the lights, alarm, door/window locks). The *order is same each day.*

These routines should be done *without exception.* These examples are illustrated in the survivor workbook.

Two basic methods to establish memory routines are outlined in the survivor workbook. One is a "memory place" such as the same parking space or key hook we just described. The other is pairing the memory routine with an already established routine or activity. This "pairing of habit" is one way to help initiate and consolidate a new routine. Review this with the survivor to identify if any helpful memory routines can be established. Use the worksheet in Visit 4 of the survivor workbook to aid this process.

Homework

- The homework is to select which of the external strategies is to be used and in what situations. Remember, your task is not to overwhelm the survivor with learning and using all compensatory strategies. Rather, select use the ones with most relevance to daily life.

- Read Visit 4 in the survivor workbook to reinforce learning and read ahead for Visit 5 if preferred.

Visit 5

Agenda and Clinician Checklist

1. *Review of Keeping a Schedule and Memory Routines*
___ Ask about what strategies were used, for what, when, where.
___ Modify as needed.
2. *External Strategies: External Cueing and Distraction Reduction*
___ External cueing rationale, brief explanation on simplified use; follow guidelines in survivor workbook sections on this topic.
___ Distraction reduction rationale, brief explanation how multitasking adversely affects learning of new information.
___ Review distraction reduction methods: auditory distractions, visual distractions, turning off electronic devices, and limiting social media use; reference survivor workbook.
3. *Activity Scheduling and Pacing*
___ Rationale for pleasant event scheduling—stress management.
___ Combined with rationale for activity pacing (scheduling an optimal amount of activity—not too much or too little).
4. *Homework*
___ Apply chosen compensatory strategy or combination.
___ Inquire about specifics of when and where strategies will be used.

Review of Keeping a Schedule and Memory Routines

- Review how the survivor is using methods of keeping a schedule or day planner and memory routines. Inquire when and where they actually use the planner and how they enter events in the planner. Is a paper day planner or an electronic device preferred? What type of planner is most practical and convenient, and which one will they actually use? How do they remind themselves to actually look at the planner and use it?

- Review which memory routines are used— is there a memory routine used with keeping a schedule (such as reviewing the day's schedule at breakfast)? Were there other memory routines with keys, personal belongings, or where they parked their car?

External Strategies: External Cueing and Distraction Reduction

External Cueing

- **External cueing** is a term referring to visual or auditory aids used as cues for important tasks (a.k.a., reminders). An example of a visual cue is a sign that reads "Wash your hands before returning to work" or a green traffic light. An example of an auditory cue is an alert in the electronic calendar on a mobile phone, or one that reminds a driver to fasten their seatbelt. The key point here is to ensure the survivor does not overuse sticky notes, alerts, or other cues that saturate the environment, because these will soon be ignored. Changing cues frequently can enhance their novelty and salience and thus their effectiveness. See the outline in the Visit 5 section of the survivor workbook to aid with instruction on this portion of external strategy.

Distraction Reduction

- **Distraction reduction** simply refers to modifying or minimizing visual or auditory stimuli in the task performance environment that could impair such performance. This usually means reducing or modifying noise in the environment or reducing or blocking visual stimuli that can distract the survivor from important tasks.

- Before cancer, many survivors may have performed well in noisy or visually distracting environments, this may have changed after diagnosis. Neuroscience and fMRI evidence points to brain activity changes that are associated with diminished learning performance when distracting auditory or visual stimuli compete with target information to be learned. Declarative memory (long-term) consolidation of complex concepts may suffer.[115] Pointing this out can help undergird the rationale for trying distraction reduction methods in MAAT and help motivate behavior change to optimize focused attention through controlled reduction of distracting stimuli.

- In the survivor workbook, an emphasis is placed on reducing distractions from mobile electronic devices that can, if allowed, keep individuals connected to the outside world 24 hours a day, every day. Texting, social networking applications, such as Instagram, Facebook, or Twitter, and email alerts on mobile devices, pagers, and telephones all have the effect of causing thought disruption and thus can quell the thorough cognitive processing necessary for encoding and deep learning. An interesting discussion on this topic is by

Dr. Calvin Newport of Georgetown University in his book *Deep Work: Rules for Focused Success in a Distracted World*.[116] The growth of mobile technology over the first two decades of the 21st century came with a concurrent cultural expectation that, somehow, individuals are available 24 hours a day to be interrupted or called upon. This is flatly false. These devices can and should be turned off for extended periods to allow us some freedom from distraction so we can focus on more important tasks that command our full attention at the workplace, at home, or in other settings. Not to mention getting uninterrupted sleep!

The growing numbers of "distracted driving" laws enacted nationally point to the impact these devices have on driving performance. According to data collected by the National Highway Traffic Safety Administration, in 2017 there were 3,166 distracted driving–related deaths of the 34,247 fatalities on U.S. highways.[117] Make this point to the survivor, who may already be cognitively compromised in the domains of processing speed and attention with CRCI. Turning off the device in the car is advisable. We have had survivors report they prefer to drive in silence, with no radio and with mobile devices put in silent mode.

- These notions are nothing new. In 2006 the researchers Foerde, Knowlton, and Poldrack[115] demonstrated that "competing dual tasks" (or so-called multitasking) can adversely affect working memory and later declarative recall, or material stored in long-term memory. In short, distraction can affect memory acquisition of new material that can be flexibly applied in new situations. The example in the survivor workbook is on applying a new vocabulary word in different contexts. Another example is applying a new computer skill to different work tasks. The authors hypothesize that medial temporal lobe systems enhance declarative learning while the striatum is used in "habit" or repetitive learning. These systems may "compete" with one another in new learning, and when a distraction is introduced, this can lead to less medial temporal activation. Obviously, this level of detail may not be necessary to discuss with the survivor, but it does point to the importance of maintaining a work or performance environment that minimizes distraction—especially for those who have cognitive complaints associated with CRCI.

- Distraction reduction methods outlined in the Visit 5 section of the survivor workbook basically involve shutting off extraneous noise or visual stimuli in the immediate environment (e.g., closing doors, windows, or blinds; turning down/off electronic music or communication devices) or wearing partial or complete noise-blocking earplugs (musicians' earplugs or sound-eliminating ear protection). Specific strategies in the survivor workbook include auditory distractions, work area auditory distractions, social setting auditory distractions, texting, mobile device alerts, and visual distractions.

Social Media Use and Distraction

- While digital connectedness through Instagram, Facebook, or Twitter social networking sites may improve social well-being in some cases, problematic social media use may lead to negative psychological consequences. Problematic social media use can be described as behaviors similar to substance use disorders, such as preoccupation with the platforms when not in use and modification of mood while using the sites. People with problematic social media use may have conflict with others about their use and may experience withdrawal symptoms when trying to quit.[118] Passive scrolling through social media content (rather than posting) and engaging in social comparison—comparing one's daily life to the positive, joyous events commonly portrayed on social media—leads to increased depression and reduced well-being.[119,120] Depressed mood is known to diminish cognitive performance, and thus making survivors aware of this process can be helpful. This is especially true with the varied and at times strong emotions associated with cancer-related social media content.

  Ask the survivor about their social media use and consider having them limit their use; in particular, they should limit passive scrolling time. Instagram and Facebook, for example, have optional settings that can set a time limit on each session and give a warning when the session is about to end. The settings on Apple iPhones and iPads (under "Screen Time") also have options for setting limits on certain apps. Another alternative is to try becoming a "digital hermit" by limiting the social network to family and close friends or even closing accounts altogether.

Activity Scheduling and Pacing

- Activity scheduling and pacing can play complementary or separate roles in the management of CRCI. First, activity scheduling is intended to increase behavioral activation in pleasant, positively reinforcing events through scheduling of daily pleasant events or achievement-oriented events.[121,122] This can improve mood and thus reduce potential negative effects of stress or depressive symptoms on attention and memory. Previous research on CRCI in breast cancer demonstrates activity scheduling improves memory and attention.[123] *Activity pacing* is used to help survivors self-regulate cognitive and physically demanding activity so as to better manage cancer-related fatigue that can diminish cognitive performance. That is, survivors should prevent exhaustion from building whenever possible. Fatigue for many survivors can persist well past completion of treatment and may be especially bothersome in the first year. Persistent pain, depression, inflammation, or anemia may be contributors to cancer-related fatigue, but research on fatigue continues.[124] Most certainly, fatigue can adversely affect cognition. A good guide for patients can be seen on the website of the National Cancer Institute's Office of Cancer Survivorship and "Facing Forward: Life After Cancer Treatment," a free booklet for cancer survivors and loved ones. There are useful sections on fatigue and other survivorship problems, including CRCI.

- The key point is that pacing involves taking brief rest periods during work tasks *before* the survivor perceives that fatigue is building up. The intent here is to *prevent* stress-related fatigue and exhaustion, not to react to it. Some research has suggested that during activity, pro-inflammatory cytokines[125] are released and build up imperceptibly, aggravating memory and attention problems. Thus, mixing in less intensive tasks or taking rest breaks during more intensive, goal-directed tasks can prevent cytokines from building up. Also, remind the survivor that quick relaxation is a form of pacing.

Therapeutic Note: For survivors who may be withdrawn or prone to depressive symptoms, activity scheduling will be important for mood regulation and thus improved cognitive performance. Combining activity scheduling and pacing for such individuals is likely beneficial. However, many survivors who present with CRCI are quite active in life and find it extremely challenging to keep pace with what was a long-held and familiar activity level prior to cancer. Therefore, scheduling achievement or pleasant activity may be the least of their concerns. Indeed, a great source of frustration or dysphoria for many survivors is the disruption of their social role functions and active lifestyle due to cancer-related fatigue. The rationale for pacing, therefore, is not to "give up" tasks or "slow down" but to use pacing as a strategy to minimize fatigue and CRCI symptom interference with valued work or home tasks. In other words, pacing is a strategy of performance enhancement, not performance compromise.

- In the survivor workbook it is suggested that survivors keep 0-to-10 ratings for pleasant events or achievement-oriented events. The intent of this is twofold. First, not all events that are positively reinforcing with regard to mood improvement are necessarily pleasant, but they can enhance a sense of achievement (e.g., cleaning the bathroom sink, mopping a floor, making an important phone call). Second, using a 0-to-10 scale establishes a healthy cognitive outlook and breaks an attitudinal habit of "black or white" or dichotomous thinking. Not all pleasant or achievement events are either "all pleasant/achieving or nothing." Rather, shades of gray are the rule—in fact, it is highly unlikely that anyone routinely experiences 0 or 10. Point this out in the discussion. Finally, keep in mind that these are guidelines and are not intended to be followed strictly. Simplicity is again stressed.

- An example of the rationale for activity scheduling and pacing may be:

"As you already know, stress and withdrawal from activity can lead to problems with memory and attention. One method of preventing increased stress is activity scheduling and pacing. Activity scheduling is a way of scheduling daily, pleasant, or achievement-oriented events designed to bring increased pleasure or a sense of achievement. For example, doing a small household chore such as cleaning a sink

may not be pleasant, but it is an accomplishment—perhaps a 2 or 3 on a 0-to-10 scale. This can help prevent loss of interest and depressed mood. Pleasant and achievement events can be work-related or with family or an interest or hobby."

Allow for discussion.

"Of course, scheduling too much activity can lead to exhaustion. It is important to pace your activity to prevent this. Pacing is simple: Change tasks frequently, before you feel fatigue building up. The intent is to prevent high levels of exhaustion, not to take a break after only you feel exhausted. Shift frequently from a fatigue-inducing task, such as house or outdoor work, to more sedentary activity, such as answering email, making a phone call, or checking finances. This way you are still productive. You are weaving it into how you go about daily life, not taking time out. Of course, it is OK to think of quick relaxation is a form of pacing."

Allow discussion.

- Review the following "Activity Scheduling Steps" (they are also included in the survivor workbook in the Visit 5 section). This can be combined with keeping a schedule as suggested in the steps. The point is to keep this simple. Ease of use is emphasized.

Activity Scheduling Steps

1) With your schedule, you are likely familiar with your daily routine, wake-up times, mealtimes, working hours, bedtimes. Include weekdays and weekends.
2) Schedule one pleasant activity (as short or as long as desired) a day. Schedule a backup event in case things do not go as planned. Keep it simple.
3) Schedule some quick relaxation (as short or as long as desired) perhaps once every hour— this helps with pacing.
4) Keep track of the most pleasant or achievement-oriented events. Write in a simple 0-to-10 rating next to the event in your schedule: 0 = no pleasure or achievement; 10 = most pleasure or achievement imaginable. Remember, not all events are going to be extremes of 0 or 10 in real life; most of our activity is somewhere in the middle.

Homework

- Review which strategies are relevant to the survivor and which will be applied and in what specific situations. Simplify.
- Consider turning off mobile devices for downtime. Limit social media use.
- Read the Visit 5 section in the survivor manual to reinforce what has been learned in this visit, but also feel free to read ahead.

Visit 6

Agenda and Clinician Checklist

1. *Review External Cueing, Distraction Reduction, and Activity Scheduling and Pacing*
___ Ask about what strategies were used, for what, when, where.
___ Modify as needed.
2. *Internal and External Strategy: Active Listening, Verbal Rehearsal for Socializing*
___ Rationale: reduce social avoidance due to cognitive problems.
___ Review nonverbal behaviors, summarization, and clarification.
___ Modeling, role play, and feedback.
3. *Fatigue Management and Sleep Improvement*
___ Rationale: use simple behavior change to minimize potential impact of sleep problems and fatigue on cognitive function.
___ Identify relevance to the survivor—if not a problem, survivor reviews workbook.
___ If so, review fatigue management and sleep quality improvement steps.
4. *Homework*
___ Apply active listening to social or occupational activity.
___ Combine with other pertinent strategies.

Review External Cueing, Distraction Reduction, and Activity Scheduling and Pacing

- Review application of using external cues, noting in which situations or environments they are most effective. Ensure the cue is simple and useful and does not "blend into the woodwork" and go unnoticed. Encourage moving the cue or cues occasionally, varying features (e.g., change the color of the note, position an object differently, change the alert sound). See if there are ways to gradually fade use of cues so the survivor is not dependent on them.

- Review distraction reduction methods. Are they helpful? Do they require modifications and can employers, family members, etc. help with reasonable accommodations to reduce distractions? Were alerts turned off on mobile phones or tablets? Is it advisable to reduce social media use?

- Review the survivor's ability to effectively implement activity scheduling and pacing and any perceived effect on memory and attention. The clinician should be aware of any problems or misunderstanding of the application of activity scheduling, pacing, or both. Some survivors feel stressed or anxious about not doing assigned tasks or believe activity scheduling is simply burdensome. That is not the intent of activity scheduling, and in fact, they may already be naturally scheduling too much. For instance, practicing progressive muscle relaxation daily, reading over the survivor workbook, and attending scheduled visits are valuable activities in themselves. Perhaps more importantly, is the survivor pacing well? Are they engaged in enough rest balanced with valued activity? Managing fatigue will result in managing CRCI well—this is discussed more in this visit.

Internal and External Strategy: Active Listening, Verbal Rehearsal for Socializing

Therapeutic Note: Active listening is a compensatory strategy used in MAAT to help reduce social avoidance due to cognitive difficulties. In a 2007 online survey conducted by Hurricane Voices Breast Cancer Foundation (with guidance from Drs. Ian Tannock and Janette Vardy), 62% of respondents reported that cognitive problems affected their social relationships at home and in the workplace. Many reported social avoidance due to embarrassment. Anecdotally, survivors participating in MAAT research have reported avoiding social situations because they had difficulty following conversations, especially in small groups when "cross-talk" or extraneous noise presented competing stimuli. Some have reported the perception that a room full of multiple conversations "is just noise, not conversation." The result is that they cannot follow the conversation and are embarrassed when others notice they are not keeping up and appear "lost" or "slow." Even when survivors in MAAT research have reported not withdrawing from social situations, they have often reported being more inclined to stay withdrawn from conversation when in the presence of others.

Active listening involves using basic interviewing methods, such as summarizing and clarifying what one heard, so that survivors can compensate for parts of conversation they may miss. It presents an opportunity to clarify and "verbally rehearse" the conversational point to register and encode. Verbal rehearsal also provides a strategy to help become re-engaged in previously avoided social activity. Obviously, if social avoidance or difficulty focusing on conversation is not a problem for the survivor, this strategy may be of less value to him or her and can be skipped.

- Review active listening as seen in the survivor workbook. In short, survivors are taught interviewing techniques of summarizing or clarifying statements—that is, repeating back what they believe the other party was saying. As with any good interview technique, this is done in a paraphrasing style with few words and can sometimes be accompanied by a clarifying question like, "Is that what you were saying?" Alternatively, the survivor can start the summarizing statement with, "So what I hear you saying is . . ." As with other compensatory strategies, modeling, role play (rehearsal), and feedback are helpful to learning the skill to achieve natural flow.

- A helpful resource for individual survivors is the classic guided self-help book on assertiveness, *Your Perfect Right: Assertiveness and Equality in Your Life and Relationships* (10th edition). This guide is full of instructions and illustrations in both active listening and asserting oneself for clarification in conversation. While many individuals who go through MAAT may not need to learn assertiveness skills, some may find the exercises in the book helpful.

- Three steps can be taken to aid with active listening skills in Visit 6.
  - First, review nonverbal behaviors of engaging in optimal eye contact (don't overuse it, don't stare, don't underuse it), relaxing one's muscles, and leaning forward when appropriate to convey that one is engaged in listening. Also, note the paralinguistic tone—that is, the tone of voice used to convey meanings of words. A tone that is of normal volume and "matter of fact" conveys confidence but not hostility or passivity. You can model the paralinguistic tone by first saying a plain phrase such as, *"The sun rises in the east and sets in the west,"* using a confident tone. The use the same tone to state a summarizing/clarifying active listening phrase like, *"So you said you were going on vacation in Maine."*
  - Second, review summarization. This is when the listener repeats back a summary of what they believe they heard. This serves the purpose of rehearsing the message sent. It also conveys that the receiver is actively listening and wants to ensure accuracy. It also opens the door for the speaker to clarify their point if it was misinterpreted or was not received correctly.
  - Third, review clarification. Clarification involves asking questions to make sure the listener heard the speaker's intended message. Examples include, "Did I hear you right?" or "Just to be clear, did you say . . .?" These and other examples are seen in the active listening section of the survivor workbook.

- Use modeling, role play, and feedback to make use of active listening skills with confidence in real-world settings. However, the real task of the clinician is to emphasize avoidance reduction. Even if the survivor lacks confidence, it is important to target social avoidance behavior so that fear of social "mistakes" can be extinguished. In the literature of social anxiety reduction, the key to reducing anxiety about small social interactions is to expose oneself to more social situations and to practice mastery of contending with whatever social interactions bring. This point should also be covered in the rationale.

- An example of the rationale for active listening may be as follows:

"Some survivors with memory and attention problems have trouble following conversations. This is especially true in places where there are several people, or in a crowded room with conversational distraction or 'cross-talk.' Active listening is simply repeating back what you believe someone said. It is a way of verbal rehearsal in a sense as it gives you an opportunity to repeat what was said."

- Allow discussion. Review both summarization and clarification. Rehearse with modeling, role play, and feedback if necessary, modeling both nonverbal and paralinguistic tone behaviors of active listening.

Fatigue Management and Sleep Improvement

- While activity pacing was covered in MAAT Visit 5, in this visit we direct more attention to fatigue management, along with discussion about improvement in sleep quality. This is especially important for survivors with CRCI, chronic fatigue, and sleep difficulty. Entire behavioral treatment programs have been developed to improve fatigue and sleep quality.[124,126] In general, fatigue during and after chemotherapy, radiation therapy, or other cancer treatments is common and can also contribute to cognitive problems.[127] Moreover, cancer survivors have higher rates of sleep difficulty compared with the general population.[128] Therefore, the goal of addressing fatigue management and sleep quality improvement is to minimize the impact of fatigue on survivors' cognitive function.

- The methods of fatigue management (including pacing, covered in Visit 5) and sleep quality improvement will not be covered in detail in MAAT, but guidelines are provided in the survivor workbook. Again, if fatigue or sleep difficulty is not an identified problem for the survivor with whom you are working, you may elect to skip this topic. However, it is worthwhile to check the relevance of these methods with each survivor. If they prefer not to cover this in detail in the visit, give them the option of simply reading about this in the survivor workbook.

- For fatigue management, there are numerous guidelines. Perhaps the most important is activity pacing. Once again, emphasize the importance of shifting from tasks requiring higher exertion to less intensive tasks based not on perceived level of fatigue *but on time or small goals.* Even if you feel full of energy, stop. Rest or do a sedentary activity, or quick relaxation. Encourage the survivor to plan ahead and communicate to well-meaning loved ones or friends to be sensitive to the survivor's plan to stop activity and not "push it." For example, the survivor could ask others ahead of time that if they make plans for the day, they should provide options for breaks or bowing out of one of the day's activities altogether. By doing so, the survivor will likely in the long run have more energy. The steps for improved fatigue management covered in the survivor workbook are detailed as follows:
  1) **Use the pacing methods outlined in the section on activity scheduling.** Breaking up daily tasks into smaller tasks and taking brief breaks will help prevent fatigue from building up. It is important to shift tasks at scheduled times even if you don't feel fatigued. This way, you will likely spread out your valued and busy activity over time and still achieve your goals but with better control of fatigue.

2) **Use relaxation skills.** In particular, be sure to practice quick relaxation through the day—this will help restore energy. Again, don't wait until you are tired or run down; do this at predetermined times.

3) **Take part in sensible exercise.** Many people who have fatigue problems avoid exercise or physical activity thinking it will add to fatigue. In fact, exercise such as walking 30 minutes a day, three or four days per week, can boost energy levels, especially if you pace yourself well. As usual, before beginning any exercise, check with your doctor or health professional. If you are not sure what type of exercise to do, many medical centers have physical therapists or personal trainers in wellness programs who can make good recommendations.

4) **Diet.** Check with a dietitian to see if there are foods you should consume more of to boost energy or if there are foods to avoid that may contribute to fatigue.

5) **Medicines, supplements, or natural substances.** Check with your doctor to see if there are safe medicines that may help with fatigue. Provigil can help with daytime fatigue and may be helpful with cognitive problems. However, medicine may not be for everyone, and there may be other supplements, vitamins, or natural ingredients that can be helpful. As always, alert your health professionals about anything you are taking: Although natural substances are "natural," they are not natural to your body and may interact dangerously with medicines.

- With respect to exercise, be sure survivors have the approval of their physician or primary care provider. Sensible, simple exercise such as walking, even if broken up through the day for short bursts, can aid with fatigue management. A website for more fatigue and sleep quality management strategies has been created by the Office of Cancer Survivorship of the National Cancer Institute (see the survivor workbook). The "Facing Forward" series can be seen online or can be downloaded as a PDF file or mailed in hardcopy form to the survivor for free.

- To improve sleep quality, see the steps outlined for stimulus control in the survivor workbook, as follows. Stimulus control is not a term you necessarily have to discuss with the survivor, but it refers to modifying the sleep environment so that the bed becomes a stimulus primarily for sleep and sexual activity but nothing else. Worry and anxious arousal in bed, especially worry about not sleeping, builds an association with the act of going to bed. Therefore, minimizing other activity in bed (e.g., worry, television watching, electronic devices with blue light, listening to music, or prolonged reading) can help build a healthy bed–sleep association. Be familiar with the points outlined in the steps for improved sleep quality.

1) **The bedroom should be a "dedicated sleep chamber."** Your bedroom or sleep area should be free of wakeful distractions. This is key since the overall goal of these steps is to increase the time spent in bed asleep and not awake.

Lying in bed awake only conditions the brain to be awake and promotes excessive worry about not sleeping. Avoid watching television, viewing tablets or mobile phones, or listening to music. Use the bed only for sleeping. Keep it dark when going to bed.

2) **The technology-free sleep chamber.** Blue light emitted by TV, mobile phone, tablet, and computer screens suppresses production of the hormone melatonin, the hormone that helps regulate sleep and wake circadian rhythms. Ideally, these devices should not be in the bedroom. If a mobile device is used as an alarm clock, simply keep the face of the phone downward and ensure all audio alerts are off. Settings or apps on some devices can help promote sleep time. Try not to view devices 45 minutes prior to going to bed. In short, blue light may promote wakefulness in the way daylight might, so a technology-free sleep chamber is a good idea.

3) **Bed times, wake times.** Go to sleep and get up at the same time each day. Having a regular schedule is important to help your brain develop regular sleep stage cycles. However, remember that if you have slept fine for a few days and have trouble sleeping one night, it doesn't necessarily mean your whole cycle will get thrown off. Just continue the schedule as regularly as possible.

4) **Don't lie in bed awake for longer than 25 to 30 minutes.** If this happens, get up and go to another room. Then, do something that is relaxing (read, listen to music, or practice your relaxation skills) and return to bed when you feel sleepy.

5) **Avoid daytime napping.**

6) **Worry time.** If you find yourself habitually thinking about things in bed that produce anxiety, such as what you need to do the next day, start scheduling a few minutes during the day (not before bed) as your "worry time" or time to schedule things you need to do tomorrow. You may conclude you have done all you can that's within your control about the topic of worry, which is a resolution that will allow for the task of sleep.

7) **Wind-down time.** Remember that some people need more time to unwind before bed than others. If you need to, allow yourself an hour (or longer) to unwind before bed—take a bath, read, watch television. Never do work right up until bedtime. Always stop at least 30 minutes to an hour before bed.

8) **Caffeine use.** Avoid caffeinated beverages after 5 p.m.

9) **Exercise schedule: Keep it sensible.** Late-night exercise may be arousing and may make it difficult to fall asleep. However, regular exercise done earlier in the day can help to regulate nighttime sleep.

- While it is desirable to cover all points on sleep quality improvement, there may not be time. If you must prioritize, cover the points of keeping regular bed and wake times and avoiding daytime naps. This can help increase sleep efficiency (that is, the proportion of time in bed during which the survivor is actually asleep). This is a primary outcome of sleep quality improvement research. Also, remove electronic devices from the bedroom. These devices can prolong states of wakefulness, and the temptation to view them while lying in bed is great, diminishing sleep efficiency. Last, instruct individuals to get out of bed if they lie awake for more than 25 or 30 minutes. Once sleepy, return to bed. This cycle may need to be repeated. Emphasize the importance of keeping the scheduled wake and sleep times without daytime naps, even if the survivor feels tired due to prolonged wakeful periods at night. Eventually, a pattern of regular sleep/wake cycles will develop.

- For a review of behavioral and cognitive treatment of insomnia or problematic sleep among cancer survivors, see the paper by Johnson et al.[126] If insomnia is a major problem for an individual survivor, treating this in a separate episode of CBT may be necessary, or referral to a psychologist or other professional competent in CBT is appropriate.

Homework

- Review which strategies are relevant and will be applied and in what specific situations.
- Simplify. Again, the point of MAAT is not to learn and master all compensatory strategies, but to select, practice, and apply those that have most potential to help daily performance for the individual survivor.
- Read Visit 6 in the survivor manual to reinforce what has been learned in this visit, but also feel free to read ahead.

[illegible] electronic devices from the bedroom. These [illegible] of wakefulness and the length of time [illegible] while lying in bed is [illegible] diminishing sleep efficiency [illegible] awake for more than 20 or 30 minutes [illegible] This [illegible] may need to be repeated. Emphasize the importance of keeping the schedule [illegible] and sleep [illegible] [illegible] at night. [illegible] will [illegible]

[illegible]

Homework

[illegible]

Visit 7

Agenda and Clinician Checklist

1. *Review Active Listening, Verbal Rehearsal for Socializing*
___ Ask about what strategies were used, for what, when, where.
___ Modify as needed.
2. *Review Fatigue Management and Sleep Quality Improvement*
___ Ask about what strategies were used, for what, when, where.
___ Modify as needed.
3. *Internal Strategy: Visualization Strategies*
___ Rationale, review visual-auditory associations.
___ Review visualization strategies (simple visualization, name–face mnemonic, method of loci); emphasize novelty and humor to evoke emotion and deepen memory.
___ Emphasize simplicity.
4. *Homework*
___ Identify, practice, and apply relevant visualization strategies—ask survivors how they might use the strategy or strategies and how they may practice in the "real world."
___ Read Visit 7 of the MAAT survivor workbook for review.

Review Active Listening, Verbal Rehearsal for Socializing

- Review use of active listening strategies of summarization and clarification. Inquire where and under what circumstances methods were tried. Reinforce and praise effort for making attempts, not performance, at this point. Like most things, performance will improve with practice. Recall one important point from Visit 6, reducing social avoidance. Even if the survivor did not absorb all content of social discussions or had word-finding difficulty, the point is to re-engage in usual social activity.

- If necessary, recall decatastrophizing or other cognitive restructuring methods to help examine or challenge maladaptive or self-deprecating thoughts in social interactions.

Review Fatigue Management and Sleep Quality Improvement

- Review application of fatigue management and sleep quality improvement methods if implemented by the survivor. Again, reinforce and praise effort for making attempts to use them. In general, improvement in sleep quality with behavioral methods takes some time; usually several weeks may pass before substantive improvements in sleep quality are noted.

- Problem-solve as needed, but encourage the survivor to keep using the methods and to continuously evaluate and modify as needed.

Internal Strategy: Visualization Strategies

- Visual imagery strategies are intended to improve verbal memory through eliciting visual–sensory associations to verbal information (names of objects or people). Theoretically, through recruiting multiple, alternative neural circuits using multiple sensory modalities, encoding and recall will be improved via "functional reorganization," where alternative circuits can bypass those damaged.[66] Visual–verbal associations thus help build alternative circuits through repeated use. Additionally, brain imaging research suggests that breast cancer survivors may have structural and activation changes in the frontal lobe, but imaging studies have not suggested occipital involvement.[129] Thus, invoking and recruiting circuitry in occipital regions with visualization strategies may promote compensatory effectiveness, though research is needed to test this hypothesis. For practical purposes of MAAT, visualization offers another option in the list of compensatory strategies.

- In MAAT Visit 7, three strategies are introduced: simple visualization, the name–face mnemonic, and the method of loci. We recommended discussing and reviewing the first two strategies with the survivor but using the method of loci as an exercise in the visit. This will provide survivors with a mastery experience with short-term recall and enhance motivation for applying it in everyday life. Model dialogue for the rationale for visualization may go as follows:

"Some neuroscientists believe circuitry in the brain's visual system can aid other parts of memory such as verbal memory—basically, using 'mental pictures' for words, numbers, or lists of things. It may make sense to use the visual system to work around other circuits of the brain (the frontal regions) that are often affected by cancer. Of course, practicing imagery can also aid visual memory, such as remembering a face and name combination."

- Visual imagery has been used for years. Enhancing emotional association with the visual image will deepen the memory.[130] Encourage the survivor to use humorous or exaggerated images (outlined later). Visual imagery is not intended for all memory tasks but is best suited for learning specific items of information such as lists of words, items, numbers (personal identification numbers [PINs] or phone numbers), computer passwords, or name–face associations.[131–133]

- Instructions for the visual imagery strategies used in MAAT are derived from several sources that have been used over the decades. Review the first two methods briefly with survivors and discuss how they might apply the methods. Encourage them to review the methods in the survivor workbook and apply them if they wish. However, once again, don't overwhelm the participant with too much procedural detail. Encourage them to select one visualization method and stick with it. Better to master one compensatory strategy than be mediocre at many!

- Most often, these visualization exercises can be practiced in the office with the clinician as a means of simply enhancing participants' attention to visual detail. In the real world, participants should be encouraged to simply use visual imagery as described in the survivor workbook. *Naturalistic practice can include trying to recall faces seen on television, on social networking sites, or in newspaper photos.* Also, "picturing" phone numbers and passwords in exaggerated, oversized letters or numbers can be done simply, quickly, and repeatedly with little disruption to daily activity. This simplifies practice. As usual, stress simplicity and ease with repeated practice; otherwise the method will not be used.

Simple Visual Imagery

If you want to use visual imagery to commit to memory an item such as a PIN or a computer password, make the visual image absurd or an exaggerated caricature. Encourage the survivor to make the visual image exaggerated or ridiculous.[130,132] For instance, as described in the survivor workbook, the survivor could imagine the four digits of the PIN to their ATM as humanoid numbers, standing with skinny arms and legs lined up at an ATM waiting impatiently while the first number slowly makes a transaction. The intent is to make the image memorable through evoking emotion. Again, emotions deepen memory—so make the image absurd and funny. The clinician should ask for details in a Socratic method, such as *"How is the image associated with the name (or procedural step or object)?"* or *"How does the image and name association make sense to you?"*

Even smells can be visualized. Olfaction holds strong associations with memory and emotional states—for example, recalling a flower not by its visual qualities but by its smell. Encourage survivors to use this sensory modality in "imagery." One survivor in past MAAT research has reported that the smell of daily medication helped with adherence to the medicine.

The Name–Face Mnemonic

The name–face mnemonic involves visualization to help the survivor with encoding and recall of name–face associations.[130,133] The participant is instructed to find an aspect of an individual's name that can be visualized. For example, reference 133 in the first sentence of this paragraph listed the author "Brooks." Picture a stream, with water running over the rocks in the streambed. Examine the person's face to find a prominent distinguishing feature, such as forehead or nose, and then visualize the "brook" running down the forehead and nose. Survivors can practice this at home with the exercises outlined in the survivor workbook such as practicing remembering the names and faces of people seen online or on TV, or new people they met in their community or workplace. Again, the "practice with the mundane and the meaningful" rule applies here.

Method of Loci ("The Journey")

Therapeutic Note: This strategy should be rehearsed with all survivors using the exercise below unless they prefer not to use any visual strategies. The method of loci, also termed "the journey" or "mental walk" in cognitive remediation literature,[102,133] has demonstrated efficacy as a mnemonic strategy to enhance sequential memory of words[134] and with verbal recall in older adults with age-associated memory changes.[133] Individuals with superior memory are known to use the strategy.[135] The method of loci is considered one of the oldest known mnemonic strategies, dating back to 477 B.C., and is attributed to the Greek poet Simonides.[136] Many teachers of rhetoric in ancient Greece taught the method of loci to students to help them memorize oratory because paper was scarce.[137]

- The method of loci is straightforward. It involves visualizing a highly familiar space such as the rooms on the ground level of one's home. The items to be remembered are pictured, one each, in each room. Variations can entail visualizing items on different body parts or along a route with familiar landmarks. The key is to use a highly familiar space that is easily recalled as one imagines walking through that space. The theoretical rationale for the method of loci is that the technique invokes the visual sensory system while encoding verbal information, thus "deepening" the memory by recruiting multiple systems in the encoding process. The visualization element may also bypass damaged verbal recall systems and thus use a new pathway to enhance recall (this segment here can be used as the rationale discussed with the survivor).
- As stated earlier, if the survivor believes this method could be useful, do the following exercise:

1) Have the survivor close their eyes and take you on a visual tour of their home, using the route they most often use. Have them describe what they "see" and describe five rooms or spaces. *A key point is to use a familiar image since this will be used as the "visual template" for the list of items to be remembered in the future.*

2) Next, give the survivor a list of five items to visualize—for instance, a gallon of milk, peas, carrots, a ball of twine, and duct tape. Have them visualize them as oversized and exaggerated in each room. State the items two or so seconds apart, using a deliberate tone. Say the last item with a falling inflexion to indicate it is the last item. In MAAT, we typically say the following:

   "Now that you have given me a visual tour, I am going to list five objects. Visualize them as absurd, big, or silly-looking. Put each item in each room or space starting at the entry point. Are you ready?" [Await reply.] *"OK. The items are . . . a gallon of milk . . . peas . . . carrots . . . a ball of twine . . . and some duct tape."*

3) Next, have the survivor describe what they saw, providing vivid detail about each object in each space. Then, after that is done, say, *"So what were the objects I asked you to remember?"* This will allow for some mastery experience. As you review homework with the survivor, ask them to recall the five objects. Do it again prior to ending the visit. This will likely again result in accurate recall and mastery of the visit.

Therapeutic Note: What about survivors who live in a studio apartment or a house with an open floor plan? Have them locate four or five places in the home, such as a coat rack, top of a dresser, countertops, furniture or cabinets, etc. If survivors have difficulty picturing their home, have them describe only two or three rooms or spaces. Conversely, if the participant wants to visualize 10 rooms or more, this is fine; 4 or 5 rooms is simply a guideline.

An alternative to using one's living space for the method of loci is using different body parts or a familiar route (e.g., commute to work). Either way, provide enough time for the participant to give an accurate description of the rooms or body parts. *This same "visual template" should be used each time they want to remember a list of items or procedural steps.*

Difficulty with Imagery

Some survivors struggle with using visual imagery, reporting it is hard for them to develop mental images. However, as with many skills, using visual imagery takes practice. Encourage survivors to try to follow the guidelines in the survivor workbook. If visual imagery is simply not for them, it is OK not to use it.

If a survivor has difficulty with visual imagery but wants to improve, two other exercises in the visit can be used. First, have the survivor look at and describe an object in the office—for example, a coffee cup or a telephone. Next, have the participant close their eyes and describe the object again. A second exercise is to simply have the survivor recall and describe the visual details of the face of a celebrity or famous person.

Homework

- Review which visualization strategy is most relevant and practical for the survivor. Encourage the survivor to try visualizing non-visual things like phone numbers or computer passwords or to make use of the method of loci. For example, have the survivor commit to the challenge of running several errands without using a written list. Once again, emphasize simplicity. The point of MAAT is not to learn and master all compensatory strategies but rather to select, practice, and apply those that have most practical use in daily life.

- Review Visit 7 in the survivor manual to reinforce what has been learned in this visit, but also feel free to read ahead.

Visit 8

Agenda and Clinician Checklist

1. *Review Visualization Strategies*
   ___ Ask about what strategies were used, for what, when, where.
   ___ Modify as needed.
2. *Tying It Together and Maintenance for Continued Quality-of-Life Improvement in Survivorship*
   ___ Visit 8 is not the end, but "the end of the beginning."
   ___ Emphasis is placed on maintaining skills learned in MAAT so that they become routine. Stress that cognitive performance failures of daily life will wax and wane.
   ___ Review adaptive strategies helpful to survivor and list them on maintenance plan form.
   ___ Identify day and time of monthly review of survivor workbook. Rationale: Life circumstances may change and thus strategies not thought to be useful in the past now may be useful.
   ___ Review the maintenance plan in the workbook.
3. *Discussion and Wrap-up*
   ___ Again, the "end of the beginning."
   ___ Have survivor schedule "booster" visits if preferred or advisable.

Review Visualization Strategies

- Review use of visualization strategies. Inquire where and under what circumstances the survivor tried various methods. What things were visualized? Did they "visualize non-visual things" such as computer passwords, PINs, etc.? Was any combination of methods used? Did visualization aid recall and performance in everyday tasks? Reinforce and praise effort for making attempts at visualization. Problem-solve if necessary and encourage practice on viewing everyday images in print, electronic, or video displays or in meeting new people. This can be done even if the information is trivial—the more the skill is practiced, the more useful it will be.

Tying It Together and Maintenance for Continued Quality-of-Life Improvement in Survivorship

- Visit 8 is not the end of treatment but "the end of the beginning" of using self-awareness and compensatory strategies to manage and cope with CRCI. With continued practice, these methods will be more skillfully used in daily life, especially during times of higher stress and life challenges when memory and attention problems are common.

- An emphasis is placed on "maintenance" of knowledge and skills gained—not "relapse prevention," which carries a negative connotation. It is normal for cognitive performance to wax and wane over time, along with the ebb and flow of the stressful demands of life, so the key is to have adaptive, compensatory strategies become routine.

- Next, review with the survivor all of the MAAT adaptive (or compensatory) strategies listed in Table 8.1. Evaluate which strategies or creative combinations thereof are helpful for the survivor. Complete step 1 of the maintenance plan in the Visit 8 section of the survivor workbook (also see Form 8.1). This involves listing each of the strategies the survivor has found helpful in daily life. Creating this list together will foster open discussion and dialogue about specific behavior changes that are useful in specific circumstances.

- After completing the list, identify with the survivor the day and time (be specific) on which they will review the survivor workbook each month. The reason for this is that life circumstances may change. For example, employment may change, and a job where verbal memory was once key to successful execution of job responsibilities may change to greater demands involving visual detail and visual working memory (such as transferring data from one spreadsheet to another). Therefore, adaptive strategies that the survivor hadn't used in MAAT to this point may have more relevance with life changes or new living circumstances. Different forms of memory may also be required with a new living situation (such as caring for an ill relative or elderly parent).

- Next, review with the survivor the five points of maintenance, one by one (listed here and in Visit 8 of the workbook). Engage the survivor in discussion about these points; make sure you don't do all the talking. Ask the survivor how important each step is to them and if they can think of personal illustrations of each point.
  1) **Self-evaluation.** Once a month, the survivor is encouraged to use the Memory and Attention Problem Record for perhaps two or three days. This is to keep up self-awareness of "at risk" situations where memory failures can have a negative impact. *This is particularly important if life circumstances change, such as job or family responsibilities.* Such a change may require a different form of memory (e.g., a change from verbal-auditory memory to more visual), and thus the survivor may be more vulnerable to different types of

Table 8.1 MAAT Strategies

Visit 1
- Self-awareness and monitoring of memory problems
- Progressive muscle relaxation

Visit 2
- Quick relaxation
- Self-Instructional Training

Visit 3
- Verbal and silent rehearsal
- Cognitive restructuring or challenging unhelpful thoughts, beliefs, and assumptions

Visit 4
- Keeping a schedule
- Memory routines

Visit 5
- External cueing
- Distraction reduction
- Activity scheduling and pacing

Visit 6
- Active listening
- Fatigue management and sleep improvement

Visit 7
- Visualization strategies

---

memory failure. Review with the survivor the example in the workbook of the nursing job change that illustrates this point.

2) **The importance of pacing.** Encourage more attention to sound pacing of activities, especially at times of higher stress and fatigue, which are times of greater risk for cognitive difficulties in daily life. It is at those higher-demand times when these stress management and inoculation methods are best applied. In short, emphasize "go with the stress; do not avoid it." There is good support for the effectiveness of these methods.

3) **The importance of practice.** Discuss with the survivor which compensatory strategies he or she uses in daily life—emphasize daily *use as practice.* Application of compensatory strategies *is practice.* Encourage refinement and modification of strategies, and encourage use of additional strategies, but at the same time keep it practical and simple. Finally, the survivor should not wait for memory problems to arise but should try to use the strategies as routine, daily habits.

4) **Review.** Encourage the survivor to review the MAAT strategies each month, as noted earlier in this visit. Emphasize again that while the survivor may

Form 8.1 Maintenance Plan

1. In the table below, list the adaptation strategies you prefer and use most in the left column. In the right column, indicate if you use the strategy daily and under what situations you are likely to use it (for example, work, home, or community). Review this once per month. Revise as needed.

Strategy	When Used, How Often? What Situations?

2. What day and time will you review your MAAT workbook each month?

3. Social support: Who will you use to help you keep on track? When will you use or ask your social support network for help?

routinely use some compensatory strategies but not others, life circumstances in family, job, or community can change. This may put new routines, responsibilities, or job tasks on the survivor's daily schedule, requiring different forms of memory and attention. Thus, compensatory strategies that are "skipped over" or not used at present may become more helpful in the future. Monthly review of MAAT may help the survivor identify and use new compensatory strategies that can prevent cognitive problems from arising when life circumstances change. Identify a specific day and time each month where the survivor can review the workbook (e.g., "first Sunday of each month, after dinner"). This is indicated in step 2 of the maintenance plan.

5) **The importance of social support.** Encourage survivors to use their supportive social relationships—family members or friends—to help with their MAAT maintenance. Encourage them to share the MAAT workbook with loved ones and to commit to practicing daily use of compensatory strategies, activity scheduling (of pleasant or achievement-oriented activities), or relaxation skills. Encourage the survivor to establish an exercise routine with a friend (again, with primary care or other physician approval) or engage in activities that require verbal-auditory or other forms of memory—for example, take a course together or engage in regular games requiring verbal memory, reasoning skills, and processing speed. Identified social support can be written in at the bottom of the maintenance plan in the survivor workbook.

Discussion and Wrap-up

- Emphasize that the conclusion of MAAT at Visit 8 is "the end of the beginning." Using the maintenance plan is one way to help ensure that the gains made in behavior change during the program will continue and that the survivor's performance in daily life will keep improving.

- While this is the last visit, the clinician should leave open the possibility for the survivor to visit again and perhaps schedule "booster visits" in the future. CRCI symptoms tend to be chronic and persistent. Therefore, refining methods or adjusting to new life circumstances or other health challenges, including cancer recurrence and additional treatment, may call for booster visits with the MAAT clinician.

References

1. Craske MG. *Cognitive–behavioral therapy*. American Psychological Association; 2010.
2. O'Donohue WT, Fisher JE. *General principles and empirically supported techniques of cognitive behavior therapy*. John Wiley & Sons; 2009.
3. Freeman A, Freeman S. *Cognitive behavior therapy in nursing practice*. Springer; 2005.
4. Freeman A. *Cognitive behavior therapy in clinical social work practice*. Springer; 2006.
5. de Moor JS, Mariotto AB, Parry C, Afano CM, Padgett L, Kent EE, Forsythe L, Scoppa S, Hachey M, Rowland JH. Cancer survivors in the United States: Prevalence across the survivorship trajectory and implications for care. *Cancer Epidemiol Biomarkers Prev*. 2013;22(4):561–70.
6. Siegel RL, Miller KD, Jemal A. Cancer statistics, 2019. *CA Cancer J Clin*. 2019;69(1):7–34.
7. Jemal A, Center MM, DeSantis C, Ward EM. Global patterns of cancer incidence and mortality rates and trends. *Cancer Epidemiol Biomarkers Prev*. 2010;19(8):1893–907.
8. Miller KD, Siegel RL, Lin CC, Mariotto AB, Kramer JL, Rowland JH, Stein KD, Alteri R, Jemal A. Cancer treatment and survivorship statistics, 2016. *CA Cancer J Clin*. 2016;66(4):271–89.
9. Stanton AL, Rowland JH, Ganz PA. Life after diagnosis and treatment of cancer in adulthood: Contributions from psychosocial oncology research. *Am Psychol*. 2015;70(2):159.
10. Silberfarb PM. Chemotherapy and cognitive defects in cancer patients. *Annu Rev Med*. 1983;34:35–46.
11. Ferguson RJ, Ahles TA. Low neuropsychologic performance among adult cancer survivors treated with chemotherapy. *Curr Neurol Neurosci Rep*. 2003;3(3):215–22.
12. Vardy J, Rourke S, Tannock IF. Evaluation of cognitive function associated with chemotherapy: A review of published studies and recommendations for future research. *J Clin Oncol*. 2007;25(17):2455–63.
13. Wefel JS, Kesler SR, Noll KR, Schagen SB. Clinical characteristics, pathophysiology, and management of noncentral nervous system cancer-related cognitive impairment in adults. *CA Cancer J Clin*. 2015;65(2):123–38.
14. Janelsins MC, Heckler CE, Peppone LJ, Ahles TA, Mohile SG, Mustian KM, Palesh O, O'Mara AM, Minasian LM, Williams AM, Magnuson A, Geer J, Dakhil SR, Hopkins JO, Morrow GR. Longitudinal trajectory and characterization of cancer-related cognitive impairment in a nationwide cohort study. *J Clin Oncol*. 2018;36(32):JCO2018786624.
15. Hurricane Voices Breast Cancer Foundation. *Cognitive changes related to cancer treatment: Survey results*. Concord, MA. 2007.
16. Ferguson RJ, Bender CM, McDonald BC, Root JC, Kucherer S. Cognitive dysfunction. In Feuerstein M, Nekhlyudov L, eds. *Handbook of cancer survivorship*. 2nd ed., Springer; 2018:199–225.
17. Mehnert A, Scherwath A, Schirmer L, Schleimer B, Petersen C, Schulz-Kindermann F, Zander AR, Koch, U. The association between neuropsychological impairment, self-perceived cognitive deficits, fatigue and health related quality of life in breast cancer survivors following standard adjuvant versus high-dose chemotherapy. *Patient Educ Couns*. 2007;66(1):108–18.
18. Schagen SB, van Dam FS, Muller MJ, Boogerd W, Lindeboom J, Bruning PF. Cognitive deficits after postoperative adjuvant chemotherapy for breast carcinoma. *Cancer*. 1999;85(3):640–50.
19. Bray VJ, Dhillon HM, Vardy JL. Cancer-related cognitive impairment in adult cancer survivors: A review of the literature. Paper presented at Cancer Forum 2017.
20. Bray VJ, Dhillon HM, Vardy JL. Systematic review of self-reported cognitive function in cancer patients following chemotherapy treatment. *J Cancer Surviv*. 2018;12(4):537–59.
21. Jim HSL, Phillips KM, Chait S, Faul LA, Popa MA, Lee Y-H, Hussin MG, Jacobsen PB, Small BJ. Meta-analysis of cognitive functioning in breast cancer survivors previously treated with standard-dose chemotherapy. *J Clin Oncol*. 2012;30(29):3578–87.
22. Ahles TA, Saykin AJ. Breast cancer chemotherapy-related cognitive dysfunction. *Clin Breast Cancer*. 2002;3(Suppl 3):S84–S90.

23. Jim HS, Donovan KA, Small BJ, Andrykowski MA, Munster PN, Jacobsen PB. Cognitive functioning in breast cancer survivors: A controlled comparison. *Cancer.* 2009;115(8): 1776–83.

24. Ferguson RJ, McDonald BC, Saykin AJ, Ahles TA. Brain structure and function differences in monozygotic twins: Possible effects of breast cancer chemotherapy. *J Clin Oncol.* 2007; 25(25):3866.

25. Silverman D, Dy C, Castellon S, Lai J, Pio BS, Abraham L, Waddell K, Petersen L, Phelps ME, Ganz PA. Altered frontocortical, cerebellar, and basal ganglia activity in adjuvant-treated breast cancer survivors 5–10 years after chemotherapy. *Breast Cancer Res Treat.* 2007;103(3):303–11.

26. Jenkins V, Shilling V, Deutsch G, Bloomfield D, Morris R, Allan S, Bishop H, Hodson N, Mitra S, Sadler G, Shah E, Stein R, Whitehead S, Winstanley J. A 3-year prospective study of the effects of adjuvant treatments on cognition in women with early stage breast cancer. *Br J Cancer.* 2006;94(6):828.

27. Hardy SJ, Krull KR, Wefel JS, Janelsins M. Cognitive changes in cancer survivors. *Am Soc Clin Oncol Educ Book.* 2018;38:795–806.

28. Mandelblatt JS, Small BJ, Luta G, Hurria A, Jim H, McDonald BC, Graham D, Zhou X, Clapp J, Zhai W, Breen E, Carroll JE, Denduluri N, Dilawari A, Extermann M, Isaacs C, Jacobsen PB, Kobayashi LC, Nudelman KH, Root J, et al. Cancer-related cognitive outcomes among older breast cancer survivors in the Thinking and Living With Cancer Study. *J Clin Oncol.* 2018;36(32): 3211–22.

29. Ahles TA, Saykin AJ. Candidate mechanisms for chemotherapy-induced cognitive changes. *Nat Rev Cancer.* 2007;7(3):192–201.

30. Tannock IF, Ahles TA, Ganz PA, Van Dam FS. Cognitive impairment associated with chemotherapy for cancer: Report of a workshop. *J Clin Oncol.* 2004;22(11):2233–9.

31. Kesler SR, Blayney DW. Neurotoxic effects of anthracycline- vs. nonanthracycline-based chemotherapy on cognition in breast cancer survivors. *JAMA Oncol.* 2016;2(2):185–92.

32. Troy L, McFarland K, Littman-Power S, Kelly BJ, Walpole ET, Wyld D, Thomson D. Cisplatin-based therapy: A neurological and neuropsychological review. *Psychooncology.* 2000;9(1):29–39.

33. Verstappen CC, Heimans JJ, Hoekman K, Postma TJ. Neurotoxic complications of chemotherapy in patients with cancer. *Drugs.* 2003;63(15):1549–63.

34. Branca JJV, Maresca M, Morucci G, Becatti M, Paternostro F, Gulisano M, Ghelardini C, Salvemini D, Mannelli LDC, Pacini A. Oxaliplatin-induced blood–brain barrier loosening: A new point of view on chemotherapy-induced neurotoxicity. *Oncotarget.* 2018;9(34):23426.

35. Dietrich J, Han R, Yang Y, Mayer-Pröschel M, Noble M. CNS progenitor cells and oligodendrocytes are targets of chemotherapeutic agents in vitro and in vivo. *J Biol.* 2006;5(7):22.

36. Ahles TA, Saykin AJ, Noll WW, Furstenberg CT, Guerin S, Cole B, Mott LA. The relationship of APOE genotype to neuropsychological performance in long-term cancer survivors treated with standard dose chemotherapy. *Psychooncology.* 2003;12(6):612–9.

37. Amidi A, Agerbæk M, Wu LM, Pedersen AD, Mehlsen M, Clausen CR, Demontis D, Børglum AD, Harbøll A, Zachariae R. Changes in cognitive functions and cerebral grey matter and their associations with inflammatory markers, endocrine markers, and APOE genotypes in testicular cancer patients undergoing treatment. *Brain Imaging Behav.* 2017;11(3):769–783.

38. Lind J, Larsson A, Persson J, Ingvar M, Nilsson L-G, Bäckman L, Adolfsson R, Cruts M, Sleegers K, Van Broeckhoven C, Nyberg L. Reduced hippocampal volume in non-demented carriers of the apolipoprotein E 4: Relation to chronological age and recognition memory. *Neurosci Lett.* 2006;396:23–7.

39. Buskbjerg CD, Amidi A, Demontis D, Nissen ER, Zachariae R. Genetic risk factors for cancer-related cognitive impairment: A systematic review. *Acta Oncol.* 2019;58(5):537–47.

40. Savitz J, Solms M, Ramesar R. The molecular genetics of cognition: Dopamine, COMT and BDNF. *Genes Brain Behav.* 2006;5(4):311–28.

41. Small BJ, Rawson KS, Walsh E, Jim HSL, Hughes TF, Iser L, Andrykowski MA, Jacobsen PB. Catechol-O-methyltransferase genotype modulates cancer treatment-related cognitive deficits in breast cancer survivors. *Cancer.* 2011;117(7):1369–76.

42. Yang M, Moon C. Effects of cancer therapy on hippocampus-related function. *Neural Regen Res.* 2015;10(10):1572.

43. Hariri AR, Goldberg TE, Mattay VS, Kolachana BS, Callicott JH, Egan MF, Weinberger DR. Brain-derived neurotrophic factor val66met polymorphism affects human memory-related hippocampal activity and predicts memory performance. *J Neurosci.* 2003;23(17):6690–4.

44. Moran M, Nickens D, Adcock K, Bennetts M, Desscan A, Charnley N, Fife K. Sunitinib for metastatic renal cell carcinoma: A systematic review and meta-analysis of real-world and clinical trials data. *Target Oncol.* 2019;14(4):405–16.

45. Laurent M, Brahmi M, Dufresne A, Meeus P, Karanian M, Ray–Coquard I, Blay J-Y. Adjuvant therapy with imatinib in gastrointestinal stromal tumors (GISTs)—review and perspectives. *Transl Gastroenterol Hepatol.* 2019;4:24.

46. During MJ, Cao L. VEGF, a mediator of the effect of experience on hippocampal neurogenesis. *Current Alzheimer Res.* 2006;3(1):29–33.

47. Mulder SF, Bertens D, Desar IM, Vissers KC, Mulders PF, Punt CJ, van Spronsen DJ, Langenhuijsen JF, Kessels RP, van Herpen CM. Impairment of cognitive functioning during sunitinib or sorafenib treatment in cancer patients: A cross-sectional study. *BMC Cancer.* 2014;14(1):219.

48. Tsavaris N, Kosmas C, Vadiaka M, Kanelopoulos P, Boulamatsis D. Immune changes in patients with advanced breast cancer undergoing chemotherapy with taxanes. *Br J Cancer.* 2002;87(1):21.

49. Pusztai L, Mendoza TR, Reuben JM, Martinez MM, Willey JS, Lara J, Syed A, Fritsche HA, Bruera E, Booser D, Valero V, Arun B, Ibrahim N, Rivera E, Royce M, Cleeland CS, Hortobagyi GN. Changes in plasma levels of inflammatory cytokines in response to paclitaxel chemotherapy. *Cytokine.* 2004;25(3):94–102.

50. Jones D, Vichaya EG, Wang XS, Sailors MH, Cleeland CS, Wefel JS. Acute cognitive impairment in patients with multiple myeloma undergoing autologous hematopoietic stem cell transplant. *Cancer.* 2013;119(23):4188–95.

51. Sharafeldin N, Bosworth A, Patel SK, Chen Y, Morse E, Mather M, Sun C, Francisco L, Forman SJ, Wong FL, Bhatia S. Cognitive functioning after hematopoietic cell transplantation for hematologic malignancy: Results from a prospective longitudinal study. *J Clin Oncol.* 2018;36(5):463–75.

52. Bevans M, El-Jawahri A, Tierney DK, Wiener L, Wood WA, Hoodin F, Kent EE, Jacobsen PB, Lee SJ, Hsieh MM, Denzen EM, Syrjala KL. National Institutes of Health hematopoietic cell transplantation late effects initiative: The Patient-Centered Outcomes Working Group Report. *Biol Blood Marrow Transplant.* 2017;23(4):538–51.

53. Syrjala KL, Artherholt SB, Kurland BF, Langer SL, Roth-Roemer S, Broeckel Elrod J, Dikmen S. Prospective neurocognitive function over 5 years after allogeneic hematopoietic cell transplantation for cancer survivors compared with matched controls at 5 years. *J Clin Oncol.* 2011;29(17):2397.

54. Hoogland AI, Nelson AM, Gonzalez BD, Small BJ, Breen EC, Sutton SK, Syrjala KL, Bower JE, Pidala J, Booth-Jones M, Jacobsen PB, Jim HSL. Worsening cognitive performance is associated with increases in systemic inflammation following hematopoietic cell transplantation. *Brain Behav Immun.* 2019;80:308–14.

55. DeSantis C, Howlader N, Cronin KA, Jemal A. Breast cancer incidence rates in US women are no longer declining. *Cancer Epidemiol Biomarkers Prev.* 2011;20(5):733–9.

56. Schilder CM, Seynaeve C, Beex LV, Boogerd W, Linn SC, Gundy CM, Huizenga HM, Nortier JW, Van de Velde CJ, Van Dam FS, Schagen SB. Effects of tamoxifen and exemestane on cognitive functioning: a study in postmenopausal patients with breast cancer: Results from the neuropsychological side study of the tamoxifen and exemestane adjuvant multinational trial. *J Clin Oncol.* 2010;28(8):1294–300.

57. Burstein HJ, Lacchetti C, Anderson H, Buchholz TA, Davidson NE, Gelmon KA, Giordano SH, Hudis CA, Solky AJ, Stearns V, Winer EP, Griggs JJ. Adjuvant endocrine therapy for women with hormone receptor-positive breast cancer: ASCO clinical practice guideline focused update. *J Clin Oncol.* 2019;37(5):423–38.

58. McGinty HL, Phillips KM, Jim HS, Cessna JM, Asvat Y, Cases MG, Small BJ, Jacobsen PB. Cognitive functioning in men receiving androgen deprivation therapy for prostate cancer: A systematic review and meta-analysis. *Support Care Cancer.* 2014;22(8):2271–80.

59. Gonzalez BD, Jim HS, Booth-Jones M, Small BJ, Sutton SK, Lin HY, Park JY, Spiess PE, Fishman MN, Jacobsen PB. Course and predictors of cognitive function in patients with prostate cancer receiving androgen-deprivation therapy: A controlled comparison. *J Clin Oncol.* 2015;33(18):2021.

60. Wefel JS, Vidrine DJ, Veramonti TL, Meyers CA, Marani SK, Hoekstra HJ, Hoekstra-Weebers JEHM, Shahani L, Gritz ER. Cognitive impairment in men with testicular cancer prior to adjuvant therapy. *Cancer*. 2011;117(1):190–6.

61. Ferguson RJ, Ahles TA, Saykin AJ, McDonald BC, Furstenberg CT, Cole BF, Mott LA. Cognitive-behavioral management of chemotherapy-related cognitive change. *Psychooncology*. 2007;16(8):772–7.

62. Kesler SR, Kent JS, O'Hara R. Prefrontal cortex and executive function impairments in primary breast cancer. *Arch Neurol*. 2011;68(11):1447–53.

63. McDonald BC, Conroy SK, Smith DJ, West JD, Saykin AJ. Frontal gray matter reduction after breast cancer chemotherapy and association with executive symptoms: A replication and extension study. *Brain Behav Immun*. 2013;30:S117–S125.

64. Stouten-Kemperman MM, de Ruiter MB, Boogerd W, Kerst JM, Kirschbaum C, Reneman L, Schagen SB. Brain hyperconnectivity >10 years after cisplatin-based chemotherapy for testicular cancer. *Brain Connect*. 2018;8(7):398–406.

65. Lower E, Harman S, Baughman R. Double-blind, randomized trial of dexmethylphenidate hydrochloride for the treatment of sarcoidosis-associated fatigue. *Chest*. 2008;133(5):1189.

66. Rohling M, Faust M, Beverly B, Demakis G. Effectiveness of cognitive rehabilitation following acquired brain injury: A meta-analytic re-examination of Cicerone et al.'s (2000, 2005) systematic reviews. *Neuropsychology*. 2009;23(1):20–39.

67. Wilson B. Neuropsychological rehabilitation. *Ann Rev Clin Psychol*. 2008;4:141–62.

68. Ferguson RJ, McDonald BC, Rocque MA, Furstenberg CT, Horrigan S, Ahles TA, Saykin AJ. Development of CBT for chemotherapy-related cognitive change: Results of a waitlist control trial. *Psychooncology*. 2012;21(2):176–86.

69. Ferguson RJ, Sigmon ST, Pritchard AJ, LaBrie SL, Goetze RE, Fink CM, Garrett AM. A randomized trial of videoconference-delivered cognitive behavioral therapy for survivors of breast cancer with self-reported cognitive dysfunction. *Cancer*. 2016;122(11):1782–91.

70. McDonald BC, Flashman LA, Arciniegas DB, Ferguson RJ, Xing L, Harezlak J, Sprehn GC, Hammond FM, Maerlender AC, Kruck CL, Gillock KL, Frey K, Wall RN, Saykin AJ, McAllister TW. Methylphenidate and memory and attention adaptation training for persistent cognitive symptoms after traumatic brain injury: A randomized, placebo-controlled trial. *Neuropsychopharmacology*. 2017;42(9):1766–75.

71. van Heugten CM, Ponds RW, Kessels RP. *Brain training: Hype or hope?* Taylor & Francis; 2016.

72. Lustig C, Shah P, Seidler R, Reuter-Lorenz P. Aging, training, and the brain: A review and future directions. *Neuropsychol Rev*. 2009;19(4):504–22.

73. Mateer CA, Sohlberg M. *Cognitive rehabilitation: An integrative neuropsychological approach*. Guilford Press; 2001.

74. Wilson BA. Compensating for cognitive deficits following brain injury. *Neuropsychol Rev*. 2000;10(4):233–43.

75. Wilson B. The clinical neuropsychologist's dilemma. *J Int Neuropsychol Soc*. 2005;11(04):488–93.

76. Lazarus RS. *Stress and emotion: A new synthesis*. Springer; 2006.

77. Ahles TA, Saykin AJ, McDonald BC, Schwartz GN, Kaufman PA, Tsongalis GJ, Moore JH, Saykin AJ. Longitudinal assessment of cognitive changes associated with adjuvant treatment for breast cancer: Impact of age and cognitive reserve. *J Clin Oncol*. 2010;28(29):4434–40.

78. Jung MS, Zhang M, Askren MK, Berman MG, Peltier S, Hayes DF, Therrien B, Reuter-Lorenz PA, Cimprich B. Cognitive dysfunction and symptom burden in women treated for breast cancer: A prospective behavioral and fMRI analysis. *Brain Imag Behav*. 2017;11(1):86–97.

79. Devolder PA, Pressley M. Causal attributions and strategy use in relation to memory performance differences in younger and older adults. *Appl Cogn Psychol*. 1992;6(7):629–42.

80. Payne BR, Jackson JJ, Hill PL, Gao X, Roberts BW, Stine-Morrow EA. Memory self-efficacy predicts responsiveness to inductive reasoning training in older adults. *J Gerontol B Psychol Sci Soc Sci*. 2012;67(1):27–35.

81. Ferguson RJ, Martinson AA. An overview of cognitive-behavioral management of memory dysfunction associated with chemotherapy. *Psicooncologia*. 2011;8(2/3):385.

82. Lachman ME, Weaver SL, Bandura M, Elliot E, Lewkowicz CJ. Improving memory and control beliefs through cognitive restructuring and self-generated strategies. *J Gerontol.* 1992;47(5):P293–P299.

83. Seidenberg M, Haltiner A, Taylor MA, Hermann BB, Wyler A. Development and validation of a Multiple Ability Self-Report Questionnaire. *J Clin Exp Neuropsychol.* 1994;16(1):93–104.

84. Ferrell BR, Dow KH, Grant M. Measurement of the quality of life in cancer survivors. *Qual Life Res.* 1995;4(6):523–31.

85. Wagner L, Sweet J, Butt Z, Lai J-S, Cella D. Measuring patient self-reported cognitive function: development of the functional assessment of cancer therapy-cognitive function instrument. *J Support Oncol.* 2009;7(6):W32–W39.

86. Bennett D. "Connect ME" is Maine's mantra for 90% of broadband by 2010. 2008.

87. McDonald BC, Ford JC, Flashman LA, et al. Neural substrate of working memory improvement following methylphenidate and cognitive-behavioral therapy for cognitive symptoms after traumatic brain injury (TBI). Platform presentation at the 12th World Congress on Brain Injury of the International Brain Injury Association; March 29–April 1, 2017; New Orleans, LA.

88. Freeman LW, White R, Ratcliff CG, Sutton S, Stewart M, Palmer JL, Link J, Cohen L. A randomized trial comparing live and telemedicine deliveries of an imagery-based behavioral intervention for breast cancer survivors: Reducing symptoms and barriers to care. *Psychooncology.* 2015;24(8):910–8.

89. West R. *Memory fitness over 40.* Triad Publishing; 1985.

90. Cicerone KD, Dahlberg C, Malec JF, Langenbahn DM, Felicetti T, Kneipp S, Ellmo W, Kalmar K, Giacino JT, Harley JP, Laatsch L, Morse PA, Catanese J. Evidence-based cognitive rehabilitation: Updated review of the literature from 1998 through 2002. *Arch Phys Med Rehab.* 2005;86(8):1681–92.

91. das Nair R, Cogger H, Worthington E, Lincoln NB. Cognitive rehabilitation for memory deficits after stroke. *Cochrane Database Syst Rev.* 2016;9(9):CD002293.

92. Holroyd KA, Holm JE, Hursey KG, Penzien DB, Cordingley GE, Theofanous AG, Richardson SC, Tobin DL. Recurrent vascular headache: Home-based behavioral treatment versus abortive pharmacological treatment. *J Consult Clin Psychol.* 1988;56(2):218.

93. Ferguson R, Mittenberg W. Sourcebook of psychological treatment manuals for adult disorders. In Van Hasselt VB, Hersen M, eds. *Cognitive behavioral treatment of postconcussion syndrome.* Plenum Press; 1995:615–52.

94. Glueckauf RL, Maheu MM, Drude KP, et al. Survey of psychologists' telebehavioral health practices: Technology use, ethical issues, and training needs. *Prof Psychol Res Pract.* 2018;49(3):205.

95. Hilty DM, Maheu MM, Drude KP, Hertlein KM. The need to implement and evaluate telehealth competency frameworks to ensure quality care across behavioral health professions. *Acad Psychiatry.* 2018;42(6):818–24.

96. Heuer A, Hector JR, Cassell V. An update on telehealth in allied health and interprofessional care. *J Allied Health.* 2019;48(2):140–7.

97. Ferguson RJ, Mittenberg W, Barone DF, Schneider B. Postconcussion syndrome following sports-related head injury: Expectation as etiology. *Neuropsychology.* 1999;13(4):582.

98. Ferguson RJ, McDonald BC, Chang H, Smith L. The role of symptom expectation and expectancy guided recall in self-reports of cognitive symptoms in cancer-related cognitive impairment. 7th Biennial International Cognition and Cancer Task Force Meeting; February 4, 2020; Denver, CO.

99. Lupien SJ, Fiocco A, Wan N, Maheu F, Lord C, Schramek T, Tu MT. Stress hormones and human memory function across the lifespan. *Psychoneuroendocrinology.* 2005;30(3):225–42.

100. Stigsdotter A, Bäckman L. Multifactorial memory training with older adults: How to foster maintenance of improved performance. *Gerontology.* 1989;35(5-6):260–7.

101. Neely AS, Bäkman L. Long-term Maintenance of gains from memory training in older adults: Two 3½ year follow-up studies. *J Gerontol.* 1993;48(5):P233–P237.

102. Yesavage JA, Rose TL. Concentration and mnemonic training in elderly subjects with memory complaints: A study of combined therapy and order effects. *Psychiatry Res.* 1983;9(2):157–67.

103. Xu L, Anwyl R, Rowan MJ. Behavioural stress facilitates the induction of long-term depression in the hippocampus. *Nature*. 1997;387(6632):497.

104. Andreotti C, Root JC, Ahles TA, McEwen BS, Compas BE. Cancer, coping, and cognition: A model for the role of stress reactivity in cancer-related cognitive decline. *Psychooncology*. 2015;24(6):617–23.

105. Thayer J, Hansen AL, Saus-Rose E, Johnsen BH. Heart rate variability, prefrontal neural function, and cognitive performance: The neurovisceral integration perspective on self-regulation, adaptation and health. *Ann Behav Med*. 2009;37:141–53.

106. Yesavage JA. Relaxation and memory training in 39 elderly patients. *Am J Psychiatry*. 1984;141(6):778–81.

107. Cohen RA. Yerkes–Dodson Law. In Kreutzer JS, DeLuca J, Caplan B, eds. *Encyclopedia of clinical neuropsychology*. Springer; 2011:2737–8.

108. Meichenbaum DH, Goodman J. Training impulsive children to talk to themselves: A means of developing self-control. *J Abnorm Psychol*. 1971;77(2):115.

109. Meichenbaum DH. Cognitive modification of test anxious college students. *J Consult Clin Psychol*. 1972;39(3):370.

110. Meichenbaum D. Self-instructional strategy training: A cognitive prothesis for the aged. *Hum Dev*. 1974;17(4):273–80.

111. Berkeley S. Reading comprehension instruction for students with learning disabilities. In Scruggs TE, Mastropieri MA, eds. *International perspectives (advances in learning and behavioral disabilities, vol. 20)*. Emerald Group Publishing Limited; 2007:79–99.

112. Chan LK. Promoting strategy generalization through self-instructional training in students with reading disabilities. *J Learn Disabil*. 1991;24(7):427–33.

113. Webster JS, Scott RR. The effects of self-instructional training on attentional deficits following head injury. *Clin Neuropsychol*. 1983;5:69–74.

114. Luik AI, Zuurbier LA, Hofman A, Van Someren EJ, Ikram MA, Tiemeier H. Associations of the 24-h activity rhythm and sleep with cognition: A population-based study of middle-aged and elderly persons. *Sleep Med*. 2015;16(7):850–5.

115. Foerde K, Knowlton BJ, Poldrack RA. Modulation of competing memory systems by distraction. *Proc Natl Acad Sci USA*. 2006;103(31):11778–83.

116. Newport C. *Deep work: Rules for focused success in a distracted world*. Hachette UK; 2016.

117. National Highway Traffic Safety Administration (NHTSA), US Department of Transportation. Distracted driving in fatal crashes, 2017. https://crashstats.nhtsa.dot.gov/Api/Public/ViewPublication/812700. Accessed January 6, 2020.

118. Griffiths MD, Kuss DJ, Demetrovics Z. Social networking addiction: An overview of preliminary findings. In Rosenberg KP, Feder LC, eds. *Behavioral addictions*. Elsevier; 2014:119–41.

119. Tandoc Jr EC, Ferrucci P, Duffy M. Facebook use, envy, and depression among college students: Is Facebooking depressing? *Computers Hum Behav*. 2015;43:139–46.

120. Verduyn P, Lee DS, Park J, et al. Passive Facebook usage undermines affective well-being: Experimental and longitudinal evidence. *J Exp Psychol Gen*. 2015;144(2):480.

121. Lewinsohn PM. A behavioral approach to depression. *Essential Papers on Depression*. 1974:150–72.

122. Robinson P, Wischman C, Del Vento A. *Treating depression in primary care: A manual for primary care and mental health providers*. Context Press; 1996.

123. Cimprich B. Development of an intervention to restore attention in cancer patients. *Cancer Nurs*. 1993;16(2):83–92.

124. Corbett T, Groarke A, Devane D, Carr E, Walsh JC, McGuire BE. The effectiveness of psychological interventions for fatigue in cancer survivors: Systematic review of randomised controlled trials. *Syst Rev*. 2019;8(1):324.

125. Kolak A, Kamińska M, Wysokińska E, Surdyka D, Kieszko D, Pakieła M, Burdan F. The problem of fatigue in patients suffering from neoplastic disease. *Contemp Oncol*. 2017;21(2):131.

126. Johnson JA, Rash JA, Campbell TS, Savard J, Gehrman PR, Perlis M, Carlson LE, Garland SN. A systematic review and meta-analysis of randomized controlled trials of cognitive behavior therapy for insomnia (CBT-I) in cancer survivors. *Sleep Med Rev*. 2016;27:20–8.

127. Small BJ, Jim HS, Eisel SL, Jacobsen PB, Scott SB. Cognitive performance of breast cancer survivors in daily life: Role of fatigue and depressed mood. *Psychooncology*. 2019;28(11):2174–80.

128. Bower JE. Cancer-related fatigue—mechanisms, risk factors, and treatments. *Nature Rev Clin Oncol*. 2014;11(10):597.

129. Nudelman KN, McDonald BC, Saykin AJ. Imaging brain networks after cancer and chemotherapy: Advances toward etiology and unanswered questions. *JAMA Oncol*. 2016;2(2):174–6.

130. Buchanan TW. Retrieval of emotional memories. *Psychol Bull*. 2007;133(5):761–79.

131. Tate RL. Subject review: Beyond one-bun, two-shoe: Recent advances in the psychological rehabilitation of memory disorders after acquired brain injury. *Brain Injury*. 1997;11(12):907–18.

132. Lewinsohn PM, Danaher BG, Kikel S. Visual imagery as a mnemonic aid for brain-injured persons. *J Consult Clin Psychol*. 1977;45(5):717.

133. Brooks JO, Friedman L, Pearman AM, Gray C, Yesavage JA. Mnemonic training in older adults: Effects of age, length of training, and type of cognitive pretraining. *Intl Psychogeriatr*. 1999;11(1):75–84.

134. Ross J, Lawrence KA. Some observations on memory artifice. *Psychonom Sci*. 1968;13(2):107–8.

135. Maguire EA, Valentine ER, Wilding JM, Kapur N. Routes to remembering: The brains behind superior memory. *Nature Neurosci*. 2003;6(1):90–5.

136. Yates FA. *The art of memory*. University of Chicago Press; 1966.

137. Bower GH. Analysis of a mnemonic device: Modern psychology uncovers the powerful components of an ancient system for improving memory. *Am Sci*. 1970;58(5):496–510.

Treatment Fidelity Checklists

Fidelity Checklist: Visit 1

Participant/Group: _____   Date: _____

Rate the fidelity to each visit element using the following 0-to-10 scale: 0 = no (poor) fidelity; 10 = highest fidelity possible.

1. *Introduction and MAAT Overview*

___ Name of MAAT, brief rationale, provide workbook.

___ Review of MAAT schedule (Table 1.1).

2. *Education on Memory and Attention Effects of Cancer and Cancer Treatments*

___ Roughly up to half of individuals with cancer or following treatment can experience subtle attention and memory difficulty.

___ Not everyone is affected, but those who are tend to have verbal memory and executive function problems (working memory, processing speed).

___ This can be long-lasting (years) but not progressive (not worse with time).

___ Causes are unclear, but changes in brain chemistry (chemotherapy, anti-estrogen effects of hormonal therapy), micro-blood vessel damage, and potential genetic vulnerability (APOE) are identified contributors, but more study is needed.

___ Bottom line: About half of cancer survivors may demonstrate long-term memory complaints; the exact prevalence remains unclear and causes are unknown, but compensatory strategies can lessen the negative impact on daily life.

3. *Memory Failure Reattribution: Not All Memory Failures Are Cancer-Related*

___ Common cancer-related memory problems (Table 1.2)—Ask, "do any of these match your experience?" Allow survivor to discuss experience with cognitive problems.

___ Now compare/contrast common memory problems of everyday life (Table 1.3).

___ Memory and attention failures are common, but not all are attributable to cancer, though clearly many can be.

____ **Important rationale**—Since we don't know all the causes of cancer-related memory problems, we know that factors such as stress (physiological changes), fatigue, and divided attention of busy, daily life also contribute to memory problems.

____ We can change environment, alter stress response, manage fatigue, and use compensatory strategies to minimize effects of memory failures.

____ Focus is on improving current cognitive function, not on what is "lost."

4.   *Self-Awareness and Monitoring Memory Problems*

____ Rationale: Identify environmental, affective, cognitive antecedents of memory failures in daily life ("know your 'at risk' situations").

____ Instruction for completion.

____ Not every memory failure is recorded but a sample of four or five forms for Visit 2.

5. *Progressive Muscle Relaxation (PMR)*

____ Rationale: Reduce sympathetic arousal that interferes with attention, encoding, and recall.

____ Enhance awareness of letting go of muscle tension *all the time, not just when stressed, to cultivate a lower baseline of arousal.*

____ Instructions: Flex muscles when you hear the word "now"—gentle flex, 30%.

____ Allow muscles to "drop" when told to relax.

____ Ignore the flexing command if a body part hurts—just focus on relaxing the muscle.

____ Instruct for home practice with audio recording.

6. *Homework*

____ Read MAAT workbook introduction and Visit 1—reassure it is all there.

____ Complete self-monitoring.

____ Daily PMR with audio recording.

Fidelity Checklist: Visit 2

Participant/Group: _____   Date: _____

Rate the fidelity to each visit element using the following 0-to-10 scale: 0 = no (poor) fidelity; 10 = highest fidelity possible.

1. *Review MAAT Reading, Relaxation and Quick Relaxation Review, Rehearsal*

   ____ MAAT reading questions.

   ____ Review PMR practice, ask about mindfulness of tense muscles in daily life.

   ____ Rationale, instruction, and rehearsal of quick relaxation.

2. *Review of Self-Monitoring, Effects of Context, Senses, and Memory Problems*

   ____ Review self-monitoring rationale, reinforce effort to keep records.

   ____ Identify the types of memory or attention failures (e.g., verbal-auditory, visual-attention, recall of written or auditory information, ability to follow instructions).

   ____ Identify environmental factors such as ambient noise, light, or other distractions.

   ____ Identify inner states such as emotions (anxiety, frustration, etc.), fatigue, hunger, pain, nausea.

   ____ Summarize types of memory failures, ask confirmation from survivor.

3. *Internal Strategy: Self-Instructional Training (SIT)*

   ____ Review rationale for compensatory strategies (prevent or reduce impact of the memory/attention failure in daily life).

   ____ Review rationale of SIT, model, rehearse.

   ____ Discuss real-world applications and how to practice in important and less important situations (over-rehearse).

4. *Homework*

   ____ Apply quick relaxation to everyday life—not to avoid anxiety or stress but to confront it with appropriate (not excessive) arousal.

   ____ Apply SIT in everyday tasks, even simple ones, to grow accustomed to the strategy.

Fidelity Checklist: Visit 3

Participant/Group: _____   Date: _____

Rate the fidelity to each visit element using the following 0-to-10 scale: 0 = no (poor) fidelity; 10 = highest fidelity possible.

1. *Quick Relaxation Review*

___ Ask about mindfulness and ability to relax muscles in everyday activity.

2. *Review Application of Self-Instructional Training (SIT)*

___ Review use of SIT in real-world situations; review examples of use.

___ If not used or rehearsed, identify reasons why, barriers, and modifications.

3. *Internal Strategy: Verbal Rehearsal Strategies (Verbal Rehearsal, Spaced Rehearsal, Chunking, and Rhymes)*

___ Rationale: rehearsal, spaced rehearsal, and other methods.

___ Identify examples in survivor's daily life; rehearse.

4. *Cognitive Restructuring: Realistic Probabilities and Decatastrophizing*

___ Rationale: Emotions are the product of cognitive appraisal, thought.

___ Identifying and challenging styles of thinking that maintain distress can aid emotional coping, not make the world perfect.

___ Review probability estimation.

___ Review decatastrophizing.

5. *Homework*

___ Apply chosen compensatory strategy or combination.

___ Use and evaluate probability estimation, decatastrophizing in daily life.

Fidelity Checklist: Visit 4

Participant/Group: _____   Date: _____

Rate the fidelity to each visit element using the following 0-to-10 scale: 0 = no (poor) fidelity; 10 = highest fidelity possible.

1. *Review of Verbal Rehearsal Strategies*

____ Ask about what verbal rehearsal strategies were used, for what, when, where.

____ Modify as needed.

2. *Review Realistic Probabilities and Decatastrophizing*

____ Inquire if these methods helped "rethink" memory problems or barriers.

____ Which method appeared to aid coping? How?

3. *External Strategy: Keeping a Schedule and Memory Routines*

____ Rationale for keeping a schedule, day planner.

____ Keep only one schedule organizer, day views, use pencil (if not electronic), simplify.

____ Rationale for keeping memory routines; keep it simple.

____ Combining these (routine to look at schedule or day planner *daily* to add/change tasks).

4. *Homework*

____ Apply chosen compensatory strategy or combination.

____ Ask about when and where strategies will be used.

Fidelity Checklist: Visit 5

Participant/Group: _____   Date: _____

Rate the fidelity to each visit element using the following 0-to-10 scale: 0 = no (poor) fidelity; 10 = highest fidelity possible.

1. *Review of Keeping a Schedule and Memory Routines*

___ Ask about what strategies were used, for what, when, where.

___ Modify as needed.

2. *External Strategies: External Cueing and Distraction Reduction*

___ External cueing rationale, brief explanation on simplified use; follow guidelines in survivor workbook sections on this topic.

___ Distraction reduction rationale, brief explanation how multitasking adversely affects learning of new information.

___ Review distraction reduction methods: auditory distractions, visual distractions, turning off electronic devices, and limiting social media use; reference survivor workbook.

3. *Activity Scheduling and Pacing*

___ Rationale for pleasant event scheduling—stress management.

___ Combined with rationale for activity pacing (scheduling an optimal amount of activity—not too much or too little).

4. *Homework*

___ Apply chosen compensatory strategy or combination.

___ Inquire about specifics of when and where strategies will be used.

Fidelity Checklist: Visit 6

Participant/Group: _____   Date: _____

Rate the fidelity to each visit element using the following 0-to-10 scale: 0 = no (poor) fidelity; 10 = highest fidelity possible.

1. *Review External Cueing, Distraction Reduction, and Activity Scheduling and Pacing*

___ Ask about what strategies were used, for what, when, where.

___ Modify as needed.

2. *Internal and External Strategy: Active Listening, Verbal Rehearsal for Socializing*

___ Rationale: reduce social avoidance due to cognitive problems.

___ Review nonverbal behaviors, summarization, and clarification.

___ Modeling, role play, and feedback.

3. *Fatigue Management and Sleep Improvement*

___ Rationale: use simple behavior change to minimize potential impact of sleep problems and fatigue on cognitive function.

___ Identify relevance to the survivor—if not a problem, survivor reviews workbook.

___ If so, review fatigue management and sleep quality improvement steps.

4. *Homework*

___ Apply active listening to social or occupational activity.

___ Combine with other pertinent strategies.

Fidelity Checklist: Visit 7

Participant/Group: _____   Date: _____

Rate the fidelity to each visit element using the following 0-to-10 scale: 0 = no (poor) fidelity; 10 = highest fidelity possible.

1. *Review Active Listening, Verbal Rehearsal for Socializing*

____ Ask about what strategies were used, for what, when, where.

____ Modify as needed.

2. *Review Fatigue Management and Sleep Quality Improvement*

____ Ask about what strategies were used, for what, when, where.

____ Modify as needed.

3. *Internal Strategy: Visualization Strategies*

____ Rationale, review visual-auditory associations.

____ Review visualization strategies (simple visualization, name–face mnemonic, method of loci); emphasize novelty and humor to evoke emotion and deepen memory.

____ Emphasize simplicity.

4. *Homework*

____ Identify, practice, and apply relevant visualization strategies—ask survivors how they might use the strategy or strategies and how they may practice in the "real world."

____ Read Visit 7 of the MAAT survivor workbook for review.

Fidelity Checklist: Visit 8

Participant/Group: _____   Date: _____

Rate the fidelity to each visit element using the following 0-to-10 scale: 0 = no (poor) fidelity; 10 = highest fidelity possible.

1. *Review Visualization Strategies*

___ Ask about what strategies were used, for what, when, where.

___ Modify as needed.

2. *Tying It Together and Maintenance for Continued Quality-of-Life Improvement in Survivorship*

___ Visit 8 is not the end, but "the end of the beginning."

___ Emphasis is placed on maintaining skills learned in MAAT so that they become routine. Stress that cognitive performance failures of daily life will wax and wane.

___ Review adaptive strategies helpful to survivor and list them on maintenance plan form.

___ Identify day and time of monthly review of survivor workbook. Rationale: Life circumstances may change and thus strategies not thought to be useful in the past now may be useful.

___ Review maintenance in the workbook.

3. *Discussion and Wrap-up*

___ Again, the "end of the beginning"

___ Have survivor schedule "booster" visits if preferred or advisable.

Progressive Muscle Relaxation (PMR) Protocol

For PMR, the clinician should remind participants of the following:

1. Lie as still as possible throughout the procedure. If you must move, do so but go back to lying as still as possible between flexion of muscles.
2. Do not flex any muscle until you hear the word "now."
3. Flex each muscle group gently, not too hard.
4. Do not flex muscles that hurt—just focus and relax.
5. Upon hearing the word "relax," let the muscle go completely, quickly, not a gradual release of tension.

PMR Protocol

This is progressive muscle relaxation. Get yourself in a comfortable, relaxed position, making sure your head and neck, and arms and hands, are comfortably supported. Now just close your eyes, and let yourself begin to relax.

*OK. I now want you to focus all your attention to your right hand, forearm, and upper arm. By making a tight fist, and pushing your right elbow down and back against the chair, you can flex the muscles of your right arm and hand, **now**. Feel the muscles pull, notice the tightness and hardness in those muscles, . . . and **relax**. Just let the tension go . . . feeling nothing . . . but the sensation of relaxation flowing through the muscles . . . notice the difference . . . between tension, that was there a moment ago, and relaxation flowing through the muscle now . . . feeling warm . . . calm . . . peaceful . . . and . . . relaxed (12 seconds).*

*All right, now let's have you focus on the muscles of the left hand . . . forearm . . . and upper arm. By making a tight fist, and pushing your elbow down and back against the chair, you can tense the muscles of you left upper arm, lower arm and hand, **now**. Feel the muscles pull, and notice that tension (5 seconds) . . . and **relax**. Let the tension go . . . allow the muscle to become more relaxed . . . as the tension flows out of these muscles. There is nothing for you to do . . . but just to allow the muscles to become more . . . and more . . . relaxed (12 seconds).*

*We will now focus on the muscles of your face. By wrinkling your forehead by trying to put your eyebrows together, and shutting your eyes tightly while gently clenching your jaw, you can tense the muscles of your upper face, lower face, and jaw, **now**. Notice the tightness and hardness in these muscles as they become tense and tight . . . feel the tension . . . and **relax**. Just letting the tension go . . . allow the forehead to smooth out . . . the eyelids to get heavy . . . allow the jaw . . . to drop. Just allow relaxation to flow over the muscles as they wind down . . . smooth out . . . and . . . relax. Noticing the difference . . . between tension that was there a moment ago . . . and relaxation that is flowing in now. Feeling . . . heavy . . . warm . . . and relaxed (12 seconds).*

*All right, I would like to have you now focus on the muscles of your neck. By pulling your chin forward without touching your chest . . . you can tense the muscles of your neck, **now**. Feel the muscles become tense and tight . . . notice the tension . . . and . . . **relax**. Just letting the muscles go . . . feeling the difference between tension . . . and . . . relaxation. Allowing the muscles to unwind . . . smooth out . . . and become more . . . and more . . . relaxed. Just enjoying . . . the peaceful . . . warm . . . feelings of relaxation as you go on relaxing more and more deeply . . . more . . . and . . . more . . . completely (12 seconds).*

*Now, by taking in a deep breath and holding it, while at the same time trying to put your shoulder blades together and making your stomach hard, you can tense the muscles of your upper back, chest, and stomach, **now**. Feel the muscles pull and become tense and tight . . . notice the tension and hardness in these muscles . . . and **relax**. Allowing the tension to go. Just experiencing relief as the tension flows out your body (5 seconds). There is nothing for you to do . . . but to simply enjoy . . . the deep . . . complete . . . feelings of relaxation . . . as you become more and more deeply and completely . . . relaxed (12 seconds).*

*OK. We will now focus on the muscles of your right leg. By lifting your right leg slightly off the chair by just a few inches, and turning your right foot downward and inward, you can tense the muscles of your right upper leg, lower leg, and foot, **now**. Feel the muscles pull and remain hard and tight . . . notice the tension . . . and **relax**. Just let the muscles go . . . notice . . . the difference . . . . between tension . . . and . . . relaxation. Just allowing the muscles to become more, and more . . . deeply . . . and completely . . . relaxed (12 seconds).*

*We will now focus on the muscles of the left leg. By lifting your left leg slightly off the chair, and turning your foot downward and inward . . . you can tense the muscles of your left upper and lower leg and foot, **now**. Feel the muscles pull and become hard and tight . . . notice the tension in these muscles . . . feel the tension . . . and **relax**. Just let the tension go . . . feel the muscles become more and more loose . . . heavy . . . and . . . relaxed. There is nothing for you to do, but to simply enjoy the warm . . . calm . . . comfortable feelings . . . of relaxation. Feeling peaceful . . . and relaxed (12 seconds).*

Now . . . we've relaxed the muscles of the arms and hands . . . just allow them to continue to relax (5 seconds). We relaxed the muscles . . . of the face . . . the neck . . . just allow these muscles to continue . . . to relax (10 seconds). We have relaxed the muscles of the upper back, the chest, and stomach . . . just allow these muscles to continue . . . relaxing (5 seconds). We have relaxed the muscles of the legs and feet . . . just allow these muscles now . . . to continue . . . relaxing (5 seconds). If there is any tension . . . anywhere in your body . . . just focus on that tension and allow that area . . . to smooth out . . . and . . . relax (10 seconds). Just allow yourself . . . to enjoy . . . the sensations of deep . . . warm . . . comfortable . . . relaxation. Feel the relaxation flowing . . . throughout your body . . . allow all the muscles to become smooth . . . comfortable . . . warm . . . and . . . relaxed (15 seconds). There is nothing for you to do . . . but to enjoy the sensations . . . of deep . . . complete . . . relaxation . . . (5 seconds). Just allow yourself now . . . to enjoy the peaceful . . . warm feelings of relaxation. More and more deeply, more . . . and more . . . completely . . . relaxed (15 seconds).

It is now time for you to return to your regular level of alertness. In a little while, I will count backward from 4 to 1. On the count of 4, you can begin to move your legs and feet . . . on the count of 3, you can begin to move your hands and arms, and on the count of 2 you can begin to move your neck and head. Then, on the count of 1, you can open your eyes. You will still feel relaxed, but you will feel refreshed, alert, and renewed. You might feel as though you have taken a short nap. Ready now, 4, moving your legs, your feet, beginning to feel more alert . . . 3, moving your hands and arms, feeling more and more awake, and alert, 2, moving your neck and head feeling more alert and awake, and 1, now beginning to open your eyes, and feeling alert, calm, awake and refreshed.

Survivor Workbook

Visit 1

In This Visit You Will:

- Complete the introduction to MAAT and go over the schedule in Table 1.1.
- Review memory and attention and problems associated with cancer.
- Review how self-awareness can improve memory performance.
- Learn how to self-monitor memory and attention failures so that you can anticipate problem situations and choose the most effective strategies.
- Learn about and practice Progressive Muscle Relaxation.

MAAT

The name of this program, Memory and Attention Adaptation Training (MAAT), emphasizes *adaptation*. Our aim is to have you start adapting new ways of doing things you did before cancer and cancer treatment in order to minimize the effects of ongoing memory problems. You are certainly not alone in survivorship. As of 2016, there were 15.5 million cancer survivors in the United States alone, with the number projected to grow to about 20.3 million by 2026.[1,2] So problems with memory and attention related to cancer affects many, and we hope MAAT will be of help to you. MAAT involves eight visits, each about 45-50 minutes long, once per week. The content of each visit is outlined in Table 1.1. This may vary depending on your speed and what is practical for you. You will use this workbook to guide you through the program step by step, so be sure to bring it with you to each MAAT visit. Feel free to underline or highlight parts of the text you believe are important.

Table 1.1 MAAT Schedule

Visit	Content
1	• Introduction and MAAT overview • Education on memory and attention and effects of cancer and treatment • Memory failure reattribution: Not all memory failures are cancer-related • Self-awareness and monitoring memory problems • Progressive muscle relaxation • Homework
2	• Review MAAT reading, relaxation and quick relaxation review, rehearsal • Review self-monitoring, effects of context, senses and memory problems • Internal strategy: Self-Instructional Training (SIT) • Homework
3	• Quick relaxation review • Review application of SIT • Internal strategy: verbal rehearsal strategies (verbal rehearsal, spaced rehearsal, chunking, and rhymes) • Cognitive restructuring: realistic probabilities and decatastrophizing • Homework
4	• Review of verbal rehearsal strategies • Review realistic probabilities and decatastrophizing • External strategy: keeping a schedule and memory routines • Homework
5	• Review of keeping a schedule and memory routines • External strategies: external cueing and distraction reduction • Activity scheduling and pacing • Homework
6	• Review of external cueing, distraction reduction, and activity scheduling and pacing • Internal and external strategy: active listening, verbal rehearsal for socializing • Fatigue management and sleep improvement • Homework
7	• Review active listening, verbal rehearsal for socializing • Review fatigue management and sleep quality improvement • Internal strategy: visualization strategies • Homework
8	• Review visualization strategies • Tying it together and continued quality-of-life improvement in survivorship • Discussion and wrap-up

Review of Memory and Attention Problems Associated with Cancer

The types of memory and attention problems many cancer survivors report differ among individuals and also depend on type of cancer treatment received. In this section, we will review the various memory problems that have been reported in research on cancer-related cognitive impairments (CRCI) with a general overview. Be sure to ask your clinician to clarify anything you have questions about or direct you to a reliable source of information on CRCI.

Common memory problems associated with CRCI may include inability to recall specific words or phrases just heard or read a short time before; forgetting names or phone numbers; and difficulty paying attention while taking steps through tasks and procedures (for example, steps in cooking or mechanical repair tasks). However, these problems vary from person to person. Some people report no problems with memory or attention after cancer. Others find they have entirely different problems of memory or attention, such as word finding difficulty. Typical memory and attention problems cancer survivors report after cancer are outlined in Table 1.2. These problems were identified in research on cancer patients who have undergone chemotherapy, but you may or may not find your experience matches this list. Many of these same symptoms have been reported by individuals who have undergone other forms of treatment, including hormonal therapies (endocrine therapies such as tamoxifen), radiation therapy, or surgery.

As you can see, survivors report a wide range of memory and attention problems. For example, in one scientific report that reviewed 16 different studies on memory effects of chemotherapy, the range of detected memory problems in the study varied from 0% to 75%! Overall, it is believed that roughly a quarter to about half of all people who have been diagnosed with and treated for cancer may have some decline in memory and attention abilities when objectively measured by standardized memory tests. Part of the reason for the large disagreements between the studies has to do with the fact that the researchers used different tests. Other reasons may be due to different effects of different cancers or different treatments. Regardless, the bottom line is that a large segment of cancer survivors experience memory problems. In the vast majority of cases they appear to be mild or moderate, but many survivors report that the problems disrupt daily life, as seen in Table 1.2.

Many cancer survivors report that their CRCI symptoms had a gradual onset. For example, an older survey completed by Hurricane Voices Breast Cancer Foundation revealed that 79% of the 471 patients said their symptoms came on gradually rather than suddenly. So this gradual onset of memory problems may be fairly common. About half of survivors reported that their symptoms "come and go," while the other half reported that they are "always present." Again, there is variability in the nature of the memory problems. Finally, 23% of survey respondents reported they had completed cancer treatment five years prior to taking the survey. Of these, 92%

Table 1.2 Common Attention and Memory Problems Reported by Cancer Survivors

1. Recalling names
2. Recalling things when trying hard
3. Recalling written details on a form
4. Recalling written information or things viewed on television
5. Remembering names, faces of people recently met
6. Making sense out of verbal explanations
7. Recalling what happened just a few minutes ago
8. Paying attention to what is going on in the immediate environment
9. Following what people are saying
10. Staying alert to what is going on

reported persistent problems with memory. So for some individuals with CRCI, the memory problems are long-lasting.

While we know that many cancer survivors will report memory and attention problems after receiving various forms of cancer and cancer therapy, it is not fully known why some people may experience CRCI and others may not. Moreover, there is some variability in the experience of CRCI. For instance, past studies suggest that high-dose chemotherapy may have a greater negative effect on memory. Still other research implies that reducing estrogen activity (a hormone associated with breast cancer *and* memory function) may play a role in negatively affecting attention and memory through causing a reduction in estrogen availability (for example, medicines such as Tamoxifen that block the actions of estrogen, or aromatase inhibiting medicines that block the production of estrogen, such as Arimidex). However, men naturally produce less estrogen than women but also report memory problems after chemotherapy or other cancer treatments, so estrogen reduction alone may not fully explain CRCI.

Genetic factors that may have a role in CRCI continue to be studied. One genetic marker, apolipoprotein E (APOE), appears to make some people vulnerable to memory problems after mild traumatic brain injury (or concussion) or the oxygen reduction effects of open heart surgery. People who have this genetic characteristic may also be more vulnerable to memory problems after chemotherapy. However, in recent research APOE did not appear to have much of an influence on memory function. This result is not final, as it may be that certain types of chemotherapy, radiation therapy, immunotherapy, or other treatments may affect APOE-positive individuals more than others. Further, more genetic factors may be at play with APOE in a complex interaction of factors, making the "genetic vulnerability" question a difficult one to answer.

There is a question about how chemotherapy or other things (such as injury) may change brain circuitry and how the cerebral cortex functions. The cerebral cortex is the large, outer portion of the brain largely responsible for associative learning, reasoning, and goal-directed behavior, which uses all forms of memory. One study conducted by the first author and colleagues at Dartmouth Medical School studied these possible effects in 60-year-old women who were identical twins. Because they were identical, they shared the exact same genetic makeup, and both were APOE positive. One was diagnosed and treated with chemotherapy and hormonal therapy for breast cancer; the other did not have breast cancer or any cancer treatment. Each was asked to complete a small battery of neuropsychological tests of memory and also complete a cognitive task in an MRI scanner—known as "functional MRI (fMRI)." The task they completed was a visual memory task that gets more difficult over three phases. Figure 1.1 displays images of each of the twins' brains.

Going left to right, the task gets more difficult. As shown, the shaded and darker areas indicate more activity in the cortex (measured as blood flow). The brain image on top is the twin who had chemotherapy (**A**); on the bottom is the non-cancer twin (**B**). As seen, the twin who had chemotherapy shows much greater activity in the cortex both at the simplest level of the task and at more difficult levels (moving right) than her sister. Of course, the unaffected twin (B) also shows more activity as the task gets more difficult from left to right, but far less than her sister who had cancer treatment.

Interestingly, each twin performed about the same on the task in the scanner and on the neuropsychological memory tests. The one difference between them was that the twin who had chemotherapy reported more difficulty with daily memory problems or symptoms than her unaffected twin. The conclusion of this twin study? Well, we cannot be certain, but the fact that there was more activation in the survivor's cortex while performing at the same level as her "normal" sister suggests that the breast cancer survivor's cortex is compensating for damaged associative memory circuits by "rewiring" or using more alternative circuits. That is, more brain is used to complete the same level of task performance. This might explain why many people who have undergone chemotherapy or other cancer treatments may score normally on standardized neuropsychological memory tests, but report they are different or slower, or that they "have to work harder to get the same result" when using their memory.

While research continues to use brain imaging methods, larger studies using multiple survivors have reached findings similar to the twin study.[3,4] The collection of these findings implies that the brain recovers after injury and can "rewire" new circuits to help with recovery of daily task performance.

Other factors that can negatively affect memory and attention after chemotherapy include the effects of anxiety, stress, and depressed mood. To be clear, the effects of cancer treatments such as chemotherapy are NOT solely due to these factors, so you can rest assured we are not saying that "chemofog" or CRCI is due to stress or anxiety. Past research has controlled for anxiety, stress and depressive symptoms and still we see memory performance scores that are lower in chemotherapy than non-chemotherapy cancer survivors.

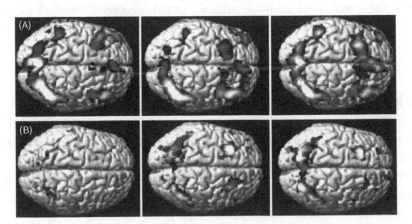

Figure 1.1 fMRI images of twins doing a memory task that gets more difficult from left to right. Note that the twin who received chemotherapy (**A**) appears to have more activation of the brain for the same task than her non-cancer twin (**B**).

Nevertheless, the impact of stress and anxiety on memory and attention function is profound. When people are stressed, anxious or have depressive symptoms, there are significant physical changes in the body that include respiration, blood flow in areas of the brain, other organs and muscles, and overall muscle tension. These responses happen to everyone under normal everyday conditions and in times of high stress. They serve the important function of helping the body deal with demands placed on it, whether these demands are from family, work, illness, or some immediate physical threat such as a wild animal attack. Basically, what the brain is trying to do is to help redirect blood, which is rich in oxygen and nutrients, to muscles in the body and critical areas of the brain— but the "thinking areas" of the brain have reduced blood flow. In someone with chronic anxiety or depressed mood (anxiety and depression that go on for a long time), the resulting changes can lead to decreased ability to focus and trouble paying attention. In turn, this interferes with the process of encoding or storing information to later be recalled as a memory. That is, problems remembering can result from information that has not been properly "stored" to begin with. Therefore, anxiety, stress and mood can negatively affect memory and attention.

Certainly, managing these problems has been studied and successful behavioral and cognitive therapies have been developed and shown to be effective in mitigating stress effects on the brain and body. While we may not fully understand the effects of the various cancer treatments on memory and attention function, we *do* know the effects of stress. This is true for everyone whether they are a cancer survivor who as undergone extensive treatment or not.

The Point of MAAT: Improve What We Know We Can

An important point needs to be made here. After reading this far, you might be wondering, "well if we know so little about this problem, how are we going to solve it?" Or, perhaps even more cynically, "why even bother?" Here is the point of MAAT: Let's focus on what is known.

We do know:

1) Various forms of cancer and cancer treatment can lead to long-term attention and memory problems for many cancer survivors.
2) These problems appear to be subtle but appear to be most bothersome for people when they begin to resume more demanding levels of work, family, and recreational activity after cancer therapy has ended.
3) These same types of problems may occur during or after other cancer treatments, such as endocrine or hormonal therapies, bone marrow transplant,

surgery, or radiation treatments, or perhaps the cancer itself. More research on all these areas is ongoing.

4) Stress, anxiety, and depression do not appear to be the sole causes of memory problems after cancer treatment. However, stress, anxiety, and depressed mood, though not a direct *cause* of memory problems, can still *contribute* and *add* to problems.

5) Often, individuals who are aware of trouble with memory and attention are understandably concerned. This concern can raise worry, and then raise the stress response. Therefore, a cycle of worry and stress can make the memory problems worse.

What we do know is how to manage the impact of memory problems on daily life *and* how to manage stress in busy 21st century life. This is what MAAT aims to help you do.

It is also important to understand that people who are healthy and who have never had any brain injury, neurological disease, or other medical conditions affecting the brain also report frequent problems with memory or attention. Indeed, often! By keeping this in mind, not *every* instance of forgetting a name, or forgetting what was spoken about in a meeting, or trouble thinking is an indication of memory disturbance. Ironically, "forgetting" actually serves an important survival function—it is the brain's way of sorting out the important from the unimportant and keeping "mental clutter" to a minimum. There is a condition called "hyperthymesia" which is characterized by being able to remember every life event in vivid detail. This is exceedingly rare, but of the few individuals with this condition, some report problems of not being able to "move on" from painful or embarrassing memories. In a sense, there is too much mental clutter getting in the way of living moment to moment.

Table 1.3 lists daily memory and attention problems reported by healthy adults. To the right of the list is the percentage of people who report experiencing the problem.

As seen, reports of different types of episodes of forgetfulness are common. *The point here is this*: if one jumps to the conclusion that every lapse in memory or attention is due to something wrong with the brain, it may only add to stress, which will indeed add to attention and memory trouble. That is, not every memory or attention lapse is completely attributable to chemotherapy or other forms of cancer treatment. Therefore, to stop this vicious cycle, keep in mind Table 1.3 and the fact that minor memory and attention problems are part of everyday healthy living. Yes, they occur in conjunction with CRCI, but cancer treatment may not be the culprit of all problems of forgetting or trouble paying attention.

To summarize:

1) We know that cancer and cancer treatment can produce problems in memory and attention. This may not be the case with every cancer survivor but those that report problems may have them for a long time.

Table 1.3 Common Things People Forget

Problem	Percent of People
Forgets telephone numbers	58%
Forgets people's names	48%
Forgets where car was parked	32%
Loses car keys	31%
Forgets groceries	28%
Forgets why they entered a room	27%
Forgets directions	24%
Forgets appointment dates	20%
Forgets store locations in shopping center	20%
Loses items around the house	17%
Loses wallet or pocketbook	17%
Forgets content of daily conversations	17%

* Source: Mittenberg W, Zielinski R, Fichera S. Recovery from mild head injury: A treatment manual for patients. *Psychotherapy in Private Practice* 1993;12:37–52.

2) At present it is not known exactly how chemotherapy or other treatments affect memory and attention function. We do know that other common factors, such as daily stress and the effects of anxiety and depression can adversely affect paying attention and remembering.

3) Keep in mind not all memory failures in daily life will be attributable to chemotherapy or cancer treatment. Some will be, but these other factors can contribute to memory failures. So, controlling what we can, such as stress reactions, being mindful by paying attention and "remembering to remember" is key.

4) In the mean time, our attempt here is to use what knowledge we have available from behavioral research to help people *cope* with and *self-manage* memory and attention problems as research continues identifying neurological processes of the problem. By focusing our energies on what we do know, and applying behavior change and memory management strategies we know can help people cope and feel more confident, the first steps can be taken to improve quality of life and management of memory problems in cancer survivorship. That is the focus of MAAT.

Types of Memory and Attention

The first part of any program that addresses problems of memory and attention involves learning more about these functions. Being familiar with different types of memory and attention can help identify your particular strengths and weaknesses and help plan strategies that play up *your* particular strengths. No one has perfect memory or is perfectly attentive all the time. In fact, one news story highlights this fact. Joshua Foer, a freelance journalist, had heard about memory championships where contestants compete at tasks such as who can be the fastest at remembering the order of a shuffled deck of cards or remembering the longest sequence of random numbers. Not only did he investigate the United States Memory Championships, but he also actually entered, trained, and set a record! However, even though he trained his memory to almost superhuman heights for competitive tasks, he still has memory failures in everyday living. "The sad truth is, I still forget where I parked my car all the time," he said in an interview with National Public Radio on February 23, 2011. "I still forget why it was that I opened the refrigerator door. I still forget to put down the toilet seat."

In summary, the strategies used to enhance memory function need to be applied to everyday life, *where memory is used*. As Mr. Foer says, "The thing about these techniques is they only work if you remember to use them. That's sort of the funny thing. You've got to remember to remember." (You can hear or read this interview archived at www.npr.org.) Knowing some basics of memory and attention can help you understand why failures in daily life such as these occur, even in memory "champions."

Attention is not just one concept of human awareness but involves some fundamental systems. Basic forms of *attention* include the following:

1) *Orientation attention*—The purpose of this form of attention is to alert us to something important; maybe a danger, a source of food, or a new and interesting object in the environment. We use orientation when we look to see where a loud noise came from.
2) *Sustained attention*—This type of attention keeps us focused on a task such as reading or listening to a teacher.
3) *Divided attention*—This form of attention enables us to split our attention for doing two things at once, such as driving while talking.
4) *Shifting attention*—This is the type of attention that lets us go from one task to another, such as stirring a pot while cooking, reading a recipe, then measuring and adding salt to the pot.

Attention is critical to *encoding*. Encoding is the process of putting new information into memory storage so that the new information can be learned and used either to carry out a task or to add to one's general knowledge. MAAT emphasizes mindfulness and attentiveness to the immediate learning task. Divided attention and distraction can detract from the process of attention and lead to reduced encoding. Since the advent of the smartphone and tablet, along with other mobile devices, the numerous distractions and interruptions these devices pose can have a detrimental effect on memory encoding. More of this is discussed in the section on distraction reduction.

As with attention, memory functions are divided among some basic systems. There are extensive writings and research on many forms of memory function that are not listed here. To help with memory in everyday life, we don't need to delve into the depths of the topic. However, here are some of the basic *memory* functions:

1) *Short-term memory*—This is memory that helps us recall things we just heard, saw, or read (within the past few minutes). An example is recalling a name of a person you just met a few minutes ago. This may also be called short-term *recall*.

2) *Long-term memory*—This is memory that allows you to remember significant things from long ago, such as a childhood memory, or things learned from a half-hour to an hour ago. This is also called long-term *recall*. A version of this that involves remembering facts, such as the date of birth of a grandparent or a historical event, is *declarative memory*.

3) *Working memory*—This is memory that allows you to hold information in your mind so you can use it to perform some act, such as going into another room to get something, or tell someone a phone number, or hearing a ZIP code and then writing it down. Working memory also helps us to remember the steps in a task, such as tying a shoe, building a birdhouse, or cooking.

4) *Recognition*—This type of memory helps you recognize things you might have forgotten; then, when you see them, you remember. A good example is when you go grocery shopping but forgot the list. At the store, you remember the items on the list because the things on the shelves remind you of items you may want. Recognition is usually easier than recall.

Again, it is not important to know these types of attention and memory functions inside and out. This is your workbook, and you can turn to this section anytime this topic comes to mind and you have a question. It is helpful to understand the basics of memory and attention systems. We know from research on the cognitive effects of cancer that many survivors report difficulty with short-term memory, working memory, recall, shifting, and divided attention. Good examples of these are listed in the prior list and in Table 1.2.

Memory and Attention Adaptation Skills

Self-Awareness and Monitoring Memory Problems

The first step in learning strategies to help aid memory and attention is to look more closely at when, where, and under what circumstances you experience memory and attention problems. As the title of this section implies, being more aware of factors that affect your memory and attention can help you prepare and do something about your memory function. Tiredness, stress, noise, emotions, and even hunger can affect memory and attention. For example, emotion can enhance memory and deepen the "network" of interconnected brain cells that store the memory. Think of where you were when you first heard the news of the attacks on New York, Washington DC, and Pennsylvania on September 11, 2001. Most people can recall what they were doing, whom they were with, and what room they were in. By contrast, try to recall what you had for lunch last Tuesday or the name of a medication you saw in an advertisement online or on television last evening. Because this probably has less emotional impact, you probably don't remember it.

Similar to emotion, the sensory systems used in establishing a memory can influence how well the memory is processed, stored, and then recalled. For example, some people, such as painters, photographers, or interior designers, are "visual." They may have an easier time picturing concepts in their minds or may remember visual features of something easier than its sound. Others are better at learning concepts with words they hear or the sounds produced by something they want to remember (such as remembering a bird species by its call rather than its appearance). Still others prefer to learn and remember things that are written, and others may remember by touch—such as the feeling of a sea shell, the wooden handle of a tool, or the texture of bread dough. Whether it is information that is seen, read, felt, or heard, the sensory system you use most will influence your attention and memory.

Keeping a brief record or "diary" of your memory and attention problems can help you discover variables that can influence them, such as emotional impact and sensory impact. Again, once you become aware of the circumstances affecting your memory and attention, you can make plans and learn skills that target your specific types of memory and attention problems. You may ask, "I already know when my memory or attention problems come up, so why should I keep a record of when this happens?" It is true that in many cases it's clear what situations can lead to trouble remembering. However, as with so much of human behavior, things that trigger problems of memory or attention may happen outside our awareness. The problems may be subtle and may differ depending on the situation. For example, some people may have trouble remembering conversations at work meetings with multiple participants but have less difficulty in social situations where they are more relaxed or with fewer people.

Form 1.1 is a memory and attention problem record. Feel free to make as many copies of this form as necessary. You should complete one record for only those memory and attention problems that bother you—those that have interfered with your work, leisure, or family life. You do not have to complete one record for each time you had trouble remembering or paying attention—that is unrealistic. But do try to sit down at least once a day and think back to situations where you had trouble remembering or paying attention. If you can, it is even better to complete one of these records as soon as possible after the problem. This helps with accuracy of details. A completed example of a record is also shown in Form 1.1.

Form 1.1 Memory and Attention Problem Record

Memory and Attention Problem Record

Date:_____ Time: _____AM PM

How much did the memory or attention problem bother you?

    0   1   2   3   4   5   6   7   8   9   10

  Not at all   Moderately   Extremely

What the memory or attention problem was:

What was happening (where you were, what you were doing, and what the surroundings were like, e.g., noisy, quiet, etc.)

What I felt at the time (Anxious? Tense? Hungry? Tired? Peaceful?

Form 1.1 Memory and Attention Problem Record EXAMPLE

Memory and Attention Problem Record

Date: *11/1/2020*   Time: _*12*_ AM (PM)

How much did the memory and attention problem bother you?

0   1   2   3   4   5   (6)   7   8   9   10

Not at all   Moderately   Extremely

What the memory or attention problem was:

Forgot the PIN to the bankcard I was using, and I also noticed it was a different card.

What was happening (where you were, what you were doing, and what the surroundings were like, e.g., noisy, quiet, etc.)

I was in the city clerk's office, and there was a line with people talking and phones ringing, confusing!

What I felt at the time (Anxious? Tense? Hungry? Tired? Peaceful?)

Felt a little rushed as many people were waiting in line. I was also hungry since I was taking care of a chore on my lunch hour.

Once you have filled out several of these forms, you can review them and look for patterns. For instance, are you having difficulty with short-term memory mostly for verbal-auditory information (words that you hear from others or from TV, radio, or online) or visual information, such as copying or transcribing telephone numbers or written materials? Alternatively, you may find that noisy environments throw off your attention or that fatigue makes it difficult to recall names. People generally vary with respect to the types of memory and attention problems they have and where and when they encounter trouble. Again, the first step in managing attention and memory problems is to improve your awareness of the situations where they are likely to arise. The next step is to target these situations and select the best strategies in this workbook to meet your particular type of memory and attention problems.

Progressive Muscle Relaxation

Another way to help with memory and attention problems is to help control the physical effects of stress. Progressive muscle relaxation (PMR) is a relaxation technique or skill that helps do this. The purpose of PMR is to help people learn to relax tense muscles and learn to better relax muscles that aren't necessary for a particular task. For instance, some people shake their leg while sitting and listening or hold a lot of tension in their shoulders. Others might find they clench their teeth while driving or grip the armrest of a chair while reading. The idea is that all that tensing takes energy and causes the nervous system to increase arousal. This increased arousal is a stress response, and this can negatively influence memory and attention. In other words, when you are relaxed, you can better focus and pay attention. And you are more likely to remember the things you pay attention to.

Becoming skilled at relaxing tense muscles takes practice. That is the downside of this exercise. On the other hand, each day, many thousands of prescriptions are written for medications that achieve the same thing. The downside of prescription medication is not only personal cost and/or side effects but also the fact that these medicines don't "teach" or "train" your nervous system to let go of tension naturally. Moreover, numerous cancer survivors who have participated in MAAT research have reported that after going through cancer treatment, they prefer not to add further medicines to their systems and would like a non-drug approach.

How It Works

Your nervous system is able to automatically run critical functions of the entire body, such as breathing, keeping the heart going to circulate blood and nutrients, and digestion, without you thinking about it. The part of the nervous system responsible for these vital functions is called the autonomic nervous system (ANS). One way to think of this is as an "auto pilot." The ANS has two branches. One activates the body and helps it escape or fight off danger when it arises. The other branch restores energy to the system and slows things down. The first branch is

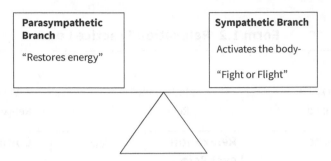

Figure 1.2 Autonomic nervous system "auto pilot."

called the sympathetic or fight-or-flight branch. This branch activates heart rate and breathing to get vital oxygen to your large muscles so you can run away or fight off danger. This is where thinking and remembering can be affected. You don't need to solve algebra problems when you're being chased by a grizzly bear. The other branch, the parasympathetic branch, will eventually kick in once the danger has passed, and it helps restore blood flow and aid digestion. It also aids sleep; this is the branch that activates after a large holiday meal and makes us sleepy. The branches counteract each other like a seesaw (Figure 1.2).

The autonomic nervous system "seesaws" throughout our lives, each day, all day, every day. While in the 21st century we do not have as many predators chasing us as our ancestors did, we retain this emergency response system, and it can create wear and tear on the body, especially if the stresses are prolonged. The key is not to avoid stress—which is impossible—but to help restore balance between the two ANS branches. One way to do this is to use relaxation techniques such as PMR. When our voluntary muscles are relaxed, we can stimulate the parasympathetic or "restoring" branch.

How To Do It

To learn to relax your muscles, you will practice a PMR exercise. The clinician will provide guidance on how to do PMR, where you will lie down and flex and relax different muscle groups, one at a time, in an exercise that will take about 15 to 20 minutes. For example, you will squeeze your right fist and gently flex the muscles of your arm for about eight seconds. Then, you will relax it. You will then move on to the other arm, then facial muscles, then legs, etc. The point of tensing and then relaxing muscle groups is to help the brain learn to let go of tension. With practice, this becomes a habit where you will let go of muscle tension almost all the time.

Your clinician or therapist may want to provide you with a practice PMR audio recording. You may also find PMR exercises that are available free of charge online. Do a simple search on "progressive muscle relaxation." Find one that suits your taste. Some people prefer music or calming nature sounds in the background, while others do not. Two suggestions are www.relaxforawhile.com or a PMR exercise found on Facebook at www.facebook/relaxforawhile. Or you may try a PMR recording at

Form 1.2 Relaxation Practice Log

0	1	2	3	4	5	6	7	8	9	10
Not At All Relaxed					Moderately Relaxed					Very Relaxed

Date	Relaxation Level Before/ After (0 to 10)	Type	Comments
___/___/___	/	☐ PMR ☐ quick	
___/___/___	/	☐ PMR ☐ quick	
___/___/___	/	☐ PMR ☐ quick	
___/___/___	/	☐ PMR ☐ quick	
___/___/___	/	☐ PMR ☐ quick	
___/___/___	/	☐ PMR ☐ quick	
___/___/___	/	☐ PMR ☐ quick	

the site for student wellness at Dartmouth College. Go to students.dartmouth.edu/wellness-center, click "Mindfulness & Meditation," and then click "Guided Audio Recordings," where you will find a recorded PMR exercise. You may also find a helpful PMR exercise on an Australian site, thiswayup.org.au/pmr-audio-2. These files can be listened to on your phone, tablet, or computer for home practice.

Form 1.2 is a log you can keep so you can see progress in your practice sessions in achieving a relaxed state. Make as many copies as you like.

When practicing PMR at home, keep the following tips in mind:

1) Lie as still as possible throughout your practice. If you must move, do so, but go back to lying as still as possible between flexion of muscles.
2) Do not flex any muscle until you hear the word "now."
3) Flex each muscle group at only about 30%.

4) Upon hearing the word "relax," let the muscle go completely and quickly rather than releasing the tension gradually.

5) If you have any muscle or mobility problems with any part of your body that makes tensing and relaxing painful (such as an injury or chronic pain), just focus and relax the area, without tension, or just tense the muscle gently. The point here is to become more mindful of letting tension go, not inducing pain. Let common sense prevail. (Individuals with lymphedema should check with their physical therapist or doctor to find out if gentle flexing is OK.)

6) You can use the relaxation log in Form 1.2 to keep track of your practice and progress. This isn't mandatory but can be helpful. The form has room for you to record your PMR practice and quick relaxation practice, another form of relaxation exercise you will learn in the next visit.

A Final Note on Visit 1 and Homework

Box 1.1 Memory and Attention Adaptation Strategies in Visit 1

- Self-awareness and monitoring of memory problems
- Progressive muscle relaxation

You have covered a lot of ground so far. You learned about some basics of memory and attention, how cancer and cancer treatments can affect memory and attention, and how other factors such as stress, emotions, and everyday activities affect these functions. You are learning two very important memory and attention adaptation strategies already: self-awareness and stress management (Box 1.1).

If you feel overwhelmed, stop. Relax. This program is designed to go at your pace. This workbook is yours to review a little at a time, at your convenience. Write notes, use a highlighter, or do whatever it takes to help you get what you want out of it. You do not have to commit to all the exercises here. Rather, take what you need and simplify and *adapt* the useful methods to your life and your activity.

To help you keep track of the strategies you try between sessions, a Homework Task Sheet is provided (Form 1.3). Just make a checkmark in the appropriate box for each day you do one of the tasks—note that there are 14 days, as sometimes you may not have weekly meetings and two weeks may elapse between visits. This form is simply to help you keep track of your practices and rehearsals in a quick and easy fashion. As you can see, there are many more things to learn as we go. But first, just focus on the tasks you need to complete before Visit 2: Complete some memory and attention problem records and practice your daily PMR. Review this visit in the workbook, and feel free to read ahead.

Form 1.3 Homework Task Sheet

Day: Homework Task	1	2	3	4	5	6	7	8	9	10	11	12	13	14
Assigned reading														
Self-awareness monitoring of memory and attention problems														
Self-Instructional Training														
Progressive muscle relaxation														
Quick relaxation														
Internal verbal rehearsal strategies (SIT, rhymes, spaced rehearsal, etc.) List here:														
External strategies (keeping a schedule, memory routine, pacing, fatigue management, etc.) List here:														

Homework Task Sheet (Example)

Day: Homework Task	1	2	3	4	5	6	7	8	9	10	11	12	13	14
Assigned reading	✓	✓	✓											
Self-awareness monitoring of memory and attention problems	✓	✓	✓	✓	✓	✓	✓							
Self-Instructional Training	✓		✓	✓			✓							
Progressive muscle relaxation														
Quick relaxation														
Internal verbal rehearsal strategies (SIT, rhymes, spaced rehearsal, etc.) List here:														
External strategies (keeping a schedule, memory routine, pacing, fatigue management, etc.) List here:														

Visit 2

In This Visit You Will:

- Review your practice and response to progressive muscle relaxation.
- Learn a new relaxation skill to help keep you relaxed in daily activity.
- Review the Memory and Attention Problem Records.
- Use your recordkeeping to help you identify useful memory strategies.
- Practice the new memory and attention strategy to apply in daily life.

Homework Review

- *Progressive muscle relaxation:* If you were able to practice the PMR exercise each day, how did the practice go in general? What muscles tended to relax the most? Did you get a sense of "letting go of muscle tension"? By contrast, which muscles stayed tense?

- If you never really achieved a sense of relaxation, don't worry: The point is practice. With practice, you will *be more mindful and aware of your tension.* You'll be more aware to achieve relaxation in everyday life while catching and letting go of tension.

- If you weren't able to practice as much as you planned, ask yourself if there is anything you can change in your schedule, or whether you ready to really give this program a good try. Either way, you have taken the first steps. Before reviewing the Memory and Attention Problem Records, let's review a shorter and perhaps more convenient relaxation exercise called quick relaxation.

Quick Relaxation

Quick relaxation is a skill that enhances your ability to quickly and effectively reduce arousal and remain calm. It involves doing brief relaxation exercises ranging from three seconds to several minutes. These quick relaxation periods are conducted dozens of times throughout the day. The idea of quick relaxation is to lower arousal before stressful events happens so that you are *optimally aroused.* That is, you are not so relaxed that you're sleepy and can't focus, but you're calmer in general. In this state, you can better focus and absorb information and may better learn it and retain it. Quick relaxation is a way to apply the effects of progressive muscle relaxation in everyday activity. Instead of waiting for the time when you listen to relaxation strategies on your smartphone or tablet, quick relaxation is designed to keep you relaxed *in the real world and in daily life.* In essence, doing many of the quick relaxation "bursts" during daily activity reminds you to stay relaxed virtually all the time. If you are mindful of maintaining optimal arousal, the inevitable stresses of everyday life can have less of a negative impact on memory and attention.

A quick relaxation exercise is done as follows:

1) First, scan your body for any tension, and focus on releasing the tension. Start at the top of your head and then focus on your neck, shoulders, arms, and each muscle down to your toes.
2) Once each muscle is more relaxed, just focus on your breathing. Do not change your breathing; just notice it. Allow your breathing to slow.
3) Each time you breathe in, say to yourself, "I am," and as you breathe out, say, "relaxed." "I am . . . ree . . . laxed." Say "relaxed" in a drawn-out manner several times. "I am . . . ree . . . laxed." Just continue for three or four more breaths. As you exhale, it is usually helpful to imagine that you are "blowing out" any muscle tension you may have. Do this repeatedly as long as you want, usually a few seconds to a minute or more. You may notice that you are more alert and focused.

You and your clinician will rehearse this quick relaxation exercise together, and you should try to apply this in daily life whenever you think of it, several times an hour or more. The point here is to cultivate optimal arousal and to be mindful and attentive to your state of arousal. Do this *before* demands on you increase arousal; don't wait until you need to respond to unexpected stressful events. Be proactive and apply this arousal regulation method in the real world.

Memory and Attention Problem Records: What Did You Find?

You and your clinician will review your Memory and Attention Problem Records in detail. In reviewing your records, you may find some trends. For instance, did you notice if the bothersome memory failures happened most at home, at the workplace, or in other settings? These questions can help you identify some *at-risk situations* where memory problems may be more likely to occur.

How about time of day? It may be that mornings at home involve busy routines of family members and yourself trying to get out the door to school or work. Also, cortisol is a stress hormone that gets released through the day. In the morning hours, it may enhance memory function and improve focus and recall. In the afternoon, where rising levels of cortisol may be less helpful, there may be a drop in memory function. So, time of day can influence memory. Morning may be your most focused time and when you feel sharpest (some studies suggest we are most productive with writing and learning in the morning). On the other hand, morning may be filled with noise, chaos, and feeling rushed to be on time, all of which can add to distraction and attention lapses. These questions can help identify time elements to your memory function.

Another dimension to consider is the *type of memory and attention problems* you have. For instance, are you having problems remembering spoken words, such as things others have said to you, what you heard in a lecture, or what you heard online or on the radio or TV? Alternatively, you might have problems with remembering what you read or saw (visual memory) or trouble following instruction steps. Finally, emotions, or feeling tired or hungry, may also influence all of these. When you get a good sense of some of the patterns of your bothersome memory failures, it will be easy to select the compensatory memory strategies that suit you best. For this visit, you'll be introduced to one of these strategies, Self-Instructional Training.

Memory and Attention Adaptation Strategies: Internal Strategies

The strategies in MAAT are "compensatory" in nature, meaning that each strategy is designed to prevent or reduce interference of the daily memory failures you may experience as a cancer survivor. MAAT consists of numerous adaptive or compensatory strategies, and you'll be introduced to and try a number of them. You will not use all that are listed in this workbook—you should experiment with strategies and select ones that fit your life and your circumstances. Internal strategies are behaviors you do "inside" yourself that others might not see, such as repeating a telephone number to yourself silently or using imagery or "mental pictures" to better remember someone's name. External strategies, in contrast, involve devices or cues in the environment that are external to you, such as keeping a schedule or day planner (discussed in Visit 4) or some sort of sign or note to remind you to do a task.

Internal and external strategy categories have been written about and studied by other cognitive rehabilitative experts such as Dr. Robin West[5] and Dr. Keith Ciscerone.[6] The first strategy you will be introduced to is an internal strategy called Self-Instructional Training.

Self-Instructional Training

Self-instructional training (SIT) is a strategy that helps improve your attention for completing tasks and remembering steps taken in tasks. It involves practicing "self-talk." That is, you will practice talking out loud to yourself when you are performing a task with many steps. By doing this, you become more aware of the individual steps and details, and this helps focus your attention. Research has shown this to be helpful

Form 2.1 Practice Form for Self-Instructional Training

Today's Date_____

Name_____   Date of Birth_____

Address

_____

_____

_____

_____

Phone Numbers

Home_____   Mobile_____

Work_____

with improving performance on many tasks for individuals who struggle with attention and short-term memory problems.

SIT involves several steps. First, your clinician will model SIT for you by talking himself or herself through a task. The task may be something you have experienced problems with, or the clinician may use the example in this workbook of filling out a form (Form 2.1). While filling out the form, the clinician might say out loud, *"Now I fill in my name on this line . . . now my address on this line"* and so forth. This is to demonstrate the strategy of self-talk by describing what they are doing.

Next, you will do the task as you talk yourself through, saying the steps out loud. You then repeat the task out loud or whisper each step. The idea is to get used to and practice self-talk in everyday, real-world situations to make your inner voice more noticeable. Eventually, you won't have to move your lips and it will become more automatic and will draw your attention to the task at hand. Repeated practice with many daily tasks can improve your focus on self-talk. Ultimately, this can improve your attention as you engage in your valued activity. By improving attention, you are more able to complete your task without missing any steps. SIT can also help improve your attention to detail. Improved attention can lead to better learning and memory storage, which means you will be more likely to recall the memory later.

Use SIT in everyday tasks. Brewing coffee, making breakfast and cleaning up, shaving, brushing your teeth, getting dressed—all these tasks involve little steps, and many of us have been sidetracked and missed a step (for example, allowing the coffee to brew but missing the step of inserting the pot in the machine!). It's important to practice SIT with "the mundane as well as the meaningful." That is, use SIT in everyday tasks so that you will be able to use it when bigger, more important tasks come your way. Of course, SIT should be applied to tasks of high difficulty such as completing a laboratory procedure with different steps, or steps in an electrical circuit board repair, or writing software code. You be the judge.

Here is a summary of the SIT practice steps:

1) Select the practice task (or you can practice filling in Form 2.1).
2) Complete the task while talking yourself through it. Be sure to include each step.
3) If you make a mistake, simply say to yourself, "OK, I was thrown off for a second. Now, let's take the next step." Mistakes are OK; just pick up where you left off.
4) After you complete the task, repeat it—only this time, whisper to yourself.
5) After that, repeat the task again, but just silently think through each step.

Homework

Box 2.1 Memory and Attention Adaptation Strategies, Visit 2

- Quick relaxation
- Self-Instructional Training

The homework to do for your next MAAT visit is to put quick relaxation into your everyday life to optimize your stress arousal and maintain calmness (Box 2.1). Be sure to use quick relaxation often, whenever and wherever you think of it. Do not wait for stress. Instead, cultivate a level of calm, always.

Next, use SIT in everyday life. You can use Form 2.1, but practice SIT with everyday tasks, always. The more you do this "self-talk," the more automatic it will become as a way to pay careful attention. Read the section covering Visit 2 in the workbook.

Visit 3

In This Visit You Will:

- Review your practice and response to quick relaxation and your overall ability to use relaxation skills in a practical way
- Review your use of Self-Instructional Training
- Review any other memory and attention problems that you've noticed
- Review strategies and select one that fits you
- Learn how to identify and challenge thinking that leads to excessive stress or erodes your emotional strength and resilience
- Practice the new memory and attention strategy by applying them in daily life

Homework Review

- *Relaxation:* How well were you able to apply quick relaxation in daily life? Are you continuing to also practice the progressive muscle relaxation once per day, or several days a week? Not all methods fit all people, so you may have by now discovered some combination of relaxation exercises that works for you.

- The key here is this: Are you becoming more *mindful and aware of tense muscles and tension in daily life? And are you able to relax muscles before they build excessive tension?* Are you using relaxation to "cultivate optimal arousal" rather than waiting to get stressed and then try to wind down? With practice, this will happen.

- Obviously, too much relaxation is not what we are emphasizing here; we don't want you to be unresponsive or sleepy! But we are emphasizing maintaining an optimal level of arousal so you perform well. This is much like a track-and-field athlete. Sprinters who have too much muscle tension usually do not run their fastest. Yes, even during a 100-meter all-out effort, world-class athletes train hours to *relax* the muscles of their upper body and jaw so that tension won't interfere with the prime objective: to move forward, fast. The aim here to keep in mind is to *relax muscles not essential for the task*. Keep up the practice you have been doing.

- *Self-Instructional Training:* Review how "self-talk" worked for you. Did it help you stay focused and on task and help you from getting sidetracked from noise such as conversations, voices, music, traffic, or other sounds? Most importantly, did you get a sense of *performing* better on daily tasks?

- Did it keep you focused visually so you weren't sidetracked by movement, objects, or reading materials? Did it help you stay focused to complete your important tasks? Did it help you avoid the temptation of glancing at email and cellphone text messages, alerts, or tweets? All of these sound and visual elements are sources of distraction.

- Remember, what you do not focus on, you will not store to memory, or you may miss a step in a task. Self-instruction (self-talk) is a helpful tool in staying "on task" and to reduce getting sidetracked. Some distractions we listed in the prior bullet are unavoidable, but some are entirely avoidable. For instance, you CAN turn off the cellphone or tablet and stow it. Minimizing distractions is discussed in "external strategies" later. For now, let's move on to more internal strategies.

Internal Strategy: Verbal and "Silent" Rehearsal

Verbal and silent rehearsal is straightforward: It simply involves repeating, silently or out loud, new information that you've just heard. The purpose of using verbal and silent rehearsal in everyday life is to improve your recall of facts, people, names, etc. Practical things may include remembering telephone numbers, addresses, or people's names so you can either recite them or write them down later.

Simple Repetition

When you hear a ZIP code, address, or name of a person you want to remember, simply repeat it out loud or silently several times, enough so you can write it down or use the information (such as dialing a phone).

Spaced Rehearsal

This is the same as verbal rehearsal but involves making the time interval slightly longer between each repetition—that is, "spacing" the intervals longer and longer between each repetition of what you're trying to remember. This method "trains" the brain to better encode or store new information. Say you want to remember a person's name. When you hear it, repeat to yourself, "Alice Jones," and then wait 3 seconds and repeat, "Alice Jones." Then wait 5 seconds and repeat, "Alice Jones," then again with an even longer interval. Visually, this would appear something like this: "Alice Jones" . . . "Alice Jones" . . . . . "Alice Jones" . . . . "Alice Jones" . . . . "Alice Jones" . . . . "Alice Jones." This method can be helpful for encoding or storing new information.

Names of People You Just Met

Forgetting the name of someone you either just met or met some time ago is quite common. It happens to many people, not only people with memory or attention problems. However, to reduce this occurrence, it is helpful to simply repeat back the name of the person you were just introduced to by looking at them, smiling, and asking to clarify if you heard the name correctly. For example, after meeting someone named Jane Jackson, you can say, "Hello. Jane Jackson? I am _____." Clarifying or repeating the person's name while looking at them helps strengthen the association between the name and the face and "deepen" the memory. You can also use this method in other social situations.

Telephone Numbers, Addresses, Etc.

Repeating back numbers either silently or out loud can help improve your memory of them, or at least help you remember until you get an opportunity to write them down. One method of helping to remember phone numbers or longer numbers is called "chunking." This involves grouping phone numbers into pairs or triplets. For example, the phone number 288-6423 can be repeated as "two eighty-eight, sixty-four, twenty-three" instead of 2-8-8-6-4-2-3. In other words, individual numbers are "chunked" into larger numbers (e.g., "6-4" becomes "64" and "2-3" becomes "23").

Whether you use verbal or silent rehearsal to remember names or numbers, daily practice and use of the strategy will yield the best results. Obviously, the best practice is when meeting new people or having someone recite a number or address to you. However, even if you have limited interactions with others, you can still practice verbal and silent rehearsal. For example, watch television news or other programs or listen to the radio and try to remember the names you hear. Also, try to remember phone numbers, addresses, or internet sites you hear on advertisements or discussed in conversation. It is sometimes a helpful exercise to memorize the mobile phone numbers of two or three of your closest loved ones rather than relying on the contacts list on your smartphone.

There are many opportunities to practice and *apply* a verbal rehearsal strategy in daily life. Do so as often as you can.

The Three Rs

Finally, a tip called the three Rs will help improve the effectiveness of silent rehearsal: Relax, Rehearse, Repeat. *Relax* your muscles and slow your breathing when listening to new information—your brain will be more receptive (quick relaxation is applicable here). *Rehearse* the new information by saying it once out loud (as in being introduced to a new person). *Repeat* the new information silently or out loud to consolidate the memory or to write it down for later use.

Rhymes

Most of us can recall nursery rhymes from childhood: "One, two, buckle my shoe . . . three, four, shut the door." The sound or "phonetic" association between similar-sounding words allows the brain to connect two bits of auditory—or word—information well. Therefore, you can use rhymes to help you remember names, numbers, or tasks to be done. The following are some examples.

Rhyming Names

This is simple with simple names, such as, "Jane from Maine," "Dan fan," "Doug on rug," etc. However, it may be a bit trickier with longer or unusual names. Don't be afraid to be creative. You may even come up with rhymes that may be unflattering to the person whose name you are trying to remember. Please don't misunderstand: We are not endorsing being cruel to others. However, adding an emotional, perhaps humorous element to the name–person association can deepen the memory and enhance its storage. For example, "Maureen the queen," "Bryant the tyrant," or "Denise has geese." Some of these rhymes may imply the opposite of their fine character or be simple nonsense, such as "Josh squash." Keep in mind that you don't have to say any of this out loud—ever!

Rhyming Tasks

A cancer survivor who was going through the MAAT program in the past indicated she had difficulty remembering the medications in her morning routine. This was critical as she also had diabetes and she needed to balance several medications to minimize complications. She came up with a rhyme that was silly but meaningful to her: "To be like Edison, take your medicine." She repeated this several times each night before going to bed as she prepared her pills for the next day. On awakening, it was nearly the first thing she said to herself. To her, it was a commonsense verbal routine that produced greater mindfulness of taking medications.

She also reported that she often forgot to take her cup of hot coffee when she left the house each morning. As it turned out, when she did her coffee routine as the last task before leaving home, she had little trouble remembering to take the coffee with her. Her rhyme? "To have a blast, coffee last." Again, silly but meaningful to her, resulting in a smoother morning routine.

Musical Rhymes

Again, this is simple. Think of the power of advertising jingles. They stick in your mind even though it's the last thing you want cluttering up your precious consciousness. What self-respecting American does not know the Roto-Rooter jingle, or any number of Coca-Cola or McDonald's songs? The point here is this: If you want to remember a name, task, or any other concept, use rhymes and put it to song. Advertisers on Madison Avenue have known this for decades. Feel free to sing it out loud (in public, at your own risk), silently, whatever. Be creative and derive meaningfulness for yourself, so use a tune you know well.

"Cognitive Restructuring" or Challenging Unhelpful Thoughts, Beliefs, and Assumptions

"It's all about attitude." "The world is what you make it." Many people are familiar with these sayings from parents, grandparents, friends, teachers, etc. While they may seem like clichés or even annoying, there is truth to each. This section provides a brief review of what clinical psychologists refer to as "cognitive restructuring" or methods to identify, challenge, and modify automatic thoughts, beliefs, or assumptions that can erode your ability to cope effectively with stress and the strong emotions that accompany it. Cognitive restructuring is a longstanding, well-researched method used in cognitive-behavioral therapies (CBTs). It is a highly effective technique used in treatment of depression and anxiety disorders as well as coping with stress produced by many chronic illnesses, including cancer.

This section will not cover cognitive restructuring in detail, so we will keep it simple. The first thing to understand is that all human emotion comes from our rapid, microsecond thoughts or perceptions. For example, if you're lying in bed in a dark room and hear a thud in the next room, you may think, "That's a burglar!" This can lead to the emotion of fear and the fight-or-flight response discussed earlier. Your heart rate, blood pressure, and breathing increase to prepare your body for the perceived threat—this is the important *function* of anxiety: to prepare! On the other hand, you might conclude that the thud was simply the dog lying down heavily on his dog bed in the next room. In this case, the thought may produce only a minor change in emotion and trigger few if any bodily reactions.

However, when you're lying in a dark room, you can only speculate or guess what caused the thud. What do you need to do to find out for sure? Go look—gather more information. That is what cognitive restructuring is: truly examining our thoughts or assumptions to come to the most accurate conclusion so that we arrive at the most appropriate or *adaptive* emotion. Notice we don't say "right or wrong emotion." All emotions serve an important survival and adaptive function—what we need for the circumstances is the most important thing. So, if a burglar were invading, fear or anger is appropriate for escape or defensive action. By contrast, fear at that level can cause unnecessary wear and tear on the body and waste energy stores if it is only the family pet lying down to rest.

Now, of course, we offer this example only to demonstrate how your thoughts or assumptions influence your emotions. It may appear to have little relationship to what you have experienced after cancer treatment. But the influence of automatic thoughts or assumptions is powerful with respect to emotional distress regarding memory problems after chemotherapy. For instance, if you assume that a failure in memory is always due to chemotherapy, then this may lead you to overlook other, more controllable factors, such as inattention when daily memory problems arise. Considering these other, more controllable factors can lead to improved coping. The key is to know *how* to examine and challenge your thinking to enhance coping in stressful moments in cancer survivorship.

How to Examine and Challenge Maladaptive or Unhelpful Thinking

The first step in examining automatic, rapid thoughts that can produce "maladaptive" or difficult-to-manage emotion is to understand just that—they are automatic and *rapid*. Most often, we have an almost instant surge of emotion (e.g., anger, anxiety), so it may be difficult to know exactly what the triggering thought was that started the ball rolling. There are numerous methods to improve our skill at identifying and challenging maladaptive thinking, but we will focus on just two in MAAT: *realistic probability estimation* and *decatastrophizing*. Appendix 2 at the end of this workbook provides more information about identifying and challenging various types of maladaptive thinking. For a more comprehensive discussion and instruction on numerous cognitive restructuring or coping methods, see the following useful books and resources:

- *Thoughts and Feelings: Taking Control of Your Moods and Your Life* by Matthew McKay, Ph.D., Martha Davis, Ph.D., and Patrick Fanning
- *The Feeling Good Handbook* by David Burns, M.D. (www.feelinggood.com)
- Association for Behavioral and Cognitive Therapies (www.abct.org)
- *Mind over Mood: Change How You Feel by Changing the Way You Think* by Dennis Greenberger, Ph.D., and Christine A. Padesky, Ph.D.

Realistic Probabilities

Research on stress and anxiety supports the idea that when we perceive a threat, we tend to make rapid judgments about whether we have the internal and external resources to cope with (overcome) the threat. For example, when anticipating a difficult exam or test in school, how well we have prepared and the degree to which we believe we mastered the course material will determine the level of anxiety or threat we feel. Sometimes, we make snap judgments about the probability of a bad outcome without considering the realities. This snap judgment can be termed "probability overestimation." That is, we may overestimate the probability that we'll do poorly on the test.

Another example is fear of flying. According to the U.S. Federal Aviation Administration, in 2019 and early 2020 there were nearly 44,000 commercial aviation flights per day in the 5.3 million miles of U.S. air space daily (faa.gov). Most years, there are no or minimal fatal commercial aviation incidents in the United States. The real probability of dying in a commercial aviation disaster is exceedingly low. According to Dr. Arnold Barnett, a professor at Massachusetts Institute of Technology who studies air traffic operations and who at one time feared flying (see: https://www.thedailybeast.com/the-great-plane-crash-myth), the actual odds of dying in the next flight one chooses to take are about 1 in 90 million—regardless of how many times one flies (or flying every day for about the next 250,000 years). Contrast that to driving an automobile: Over a lifetime of car trips (about 50,000 per person) the odds of being killed are 1 in 140, according to the National Safety Council. Given these statistics, it is irrational to fear air travel while casually getting behind the wheel and driving down the road with no apprehension whatsoever. But many do, because they overestimate the probability of dying in a plane crash.

So how do you estimate the real probability versus the "anxious" or irrational probability? It is easy when you have numerous industry or government statistics and sophisticated databases—this is one way. But how do you challenge "anxious probabilities" in daily life? One method is to do some basic mathematical estimating. Simply ask, "Of the last 10 times I have experienced (a situation), how many times did it result in (a negative outcome)?" Obviously 1 in 10 is 10%—or a 90% chance of a positive outcome. In short, simply ask yourself, "What is the REAL probability that (a negative outcome) will occur versus my 'anxious' probability?" With respect to memory failure, you might try challenging the thought that some disastrous consequence could occur if you forget a word during a presentation, or forget someone's name. For example, "What is the probability I will lose my job if I forget a word during my presentation? What is the real probability?" You may find the probability of the catastrophic consequence is far less than anticipated. A word of warning: If you say to yourself, "Yes, but . . ." after you examine the objective, estimated probability, you'll likely return to the original probability overestimating thought. Eliminate "yes, buts."

Decatastrophizing

We all know that the human tendency to overestimate the probability something bad might happen is one way to prepare, but too much overestimating negative outcomes leads to excessive anxiety. At the same time, exceedingly rare events can and do occur; planes do crash and people die; people do get rare diseases. Catastrophic events are possible. However, what do we do when that happens? Is it the end? No. It may certainly be the end of life familiar to us, and now that has changed. We may be shocked, mourn the loss, and then slowly, over time, learn to live with loss. We may never get over the loss (no such thing as "closure"), but we do live on with it somehow. In short, "decatastrophizing" is a form of accepting, but also understanding, that time and life events march onward. That is, while rare events can occur, we continue to live past and with these events.

A simple way to decatastrophize is to simply ask, "What then? And then what? And then what?" etc., etc. What this usually results in is the conclusion that after a negative event occurs, there is recovery and resumption of life. We learn that while we might not want to, we can adapt to circumstances and manage them appropriately.

For example, let's say you do lose your job because of cognitive difficulties leading to errors at work:

> "Then what? I would be angry, actually really scared. Then what? I would leave that job. Then what? I would reduce my spending, watch my budget. Then what? I would start calling colleagues or friends for other jobs. Then what? I would more than likely get one, because I have been offered others at this one place that likes my work. Then what? I would probably see what they could offer."

In summary, while bad things in life happen, we often avoid thinking through what we would actually do. Some clinicians theorize that painful thoughts of bad life events are too aversive, so we "stop" the catastrophic thought and distract ourselves with something else. The problem is that distraction doesn't allow full processing of the thought in a reasoned way, so once the distraction is done, the catastrophic thought with high emotion returns. In a sense, decatastrophizing helps us to confront these unpleasant life events and think through what we may *actually* do—which, quite likely, is to adapt.

In closing, another simple method of decatastrophizing is to simply say, "So?" For example:

> "I will look like a fool if I forget my supervisor's name at the meeting. So? What happens then if I do? Would I actually get fired?"

In addition, you may also conclude that the catastrophic event is so highly unlikely (low probability) that it is not even worth thinking about.

Homework

As usual with MAAT, the homework to do for the next visit is to try applying one of the verbal rehearsal strategies you think works best for you (Box 3.1). It is more important for you to master one strategy and become proficient with it than try several with no sense of mastery or practical help. Try memorizing two or three mobile phone numbers of loved ones or friends using your favorite verbal rehearsal method. Be practical.

Also, put into practice the thought challenge methods of probability estimation and decatastrophizing to any negative thoughts you may have about your memory problems. Practice them by applying them to the real world and in situations that you know may give you trouble. The more you practice, and even discuss with others, the easier and more effective it will be.

You can also use the homework task sheet seen in the Visit 1 section to keep track. In Appendix 2 there is more review of different thought-challenging methods and a written exercise. You can try this if you like. Review this section of the workbook, and if you wish you can read ahead for the next visit.

Box 3.1 Memory and Attention Adaptation Strategies, Visit 3

Verbal and silent rehearsal
Cognitive restructuring or challenging unhelpful thoughts, beliefs, and assumptions

Visit 4

In This Visit You Will:

- Review your practice and use of rehearsal strategies and all skills to date (relaxation, etc.).
- Be introduced to external strategies of keeping a schedule and memory routines.
- Practice the new memory and attention strategy to apply in daily life.

Homework Review

- Which methods work best for you? Is it simple verbal rehearsal, spaced rehearsal, or some combination? Does rhyming help store memory with deeper meaning, or does using melodies help? Does Self-Instructional Training have an impact or is it best used in combination with other methods?

- How about challenging maladaptive thoughts or assumptions? Does probability estimation or decatastrophizing help you cope with some of the challenges you face?

- In which situations are you most likely to use the methods? Going over these questions with your clinician will help you identify commonsense applications to improve use of your verbal working memory and attention.

External Strategies

"External strategies" refers to a set of methods that are used "outside of yourself" that may not have a direct impact on your memory and attention but can aid your memory and attention functions and avoid the pitfalls of everyday memory failures or problems associated with them.

Keeping a Schedule

The purpose of using and keeping a daily schedule is (1) to reduce the risk of becoming overwhelmed by multiple tasks and (2) to establish a regular routine to the greatest extent possible. Keeping a simplified but complete schedule can help tremendously with remembering important tasks, eliminating "to-do" lists, and freeing you from worry about missing important appointments, personal tasks, or phone calls. A good schedule is a great method of time and stress management. Surprisingly, numerous high-functioning cancer survivors do not keep an effective schedule of daily tasks. In a sense, it is as though before cancer, they did not need to keep track of personal events of work, home, and family—they were perfectly capable of keeping track of planned activity without writing it down on paper or entering it into an electronic device. However, after cancer treatment, many find that it becomes more difficult to retain and recall important events. To keep an effective daily schedule, here are suggested steps:

1) **Use a day planner.** Electronic devices such as smartphones and tablets combine communications technologies and offer a vast array of scheduling options. However, an old-fashioned paper day planner has some advantages: (1) it does not have to be charged and will not run out of battery power; (2) it requires no "set-up" time; and (3) there is no monthly fee for mobile phone or internet access. For those who like these advantages and given these upsides, buy one that has *one page for one day*. Avoid day planners with week or month displays because these do not allow enough space to write in daily tasks or appointments clearly. Conversely, hourly slots allow easy entry for tasks. Most schedules or day planners list all the daytime hours on one page, with some space devoted to evening hours:

April 5, 2021

6:00 a.m._____

7:00 a.m._____

8:00 a.m._____

9:00 a.m._____

10:00 a.m._____

11:00 a.m._____

Noon_____

1:00 p.m._____

2:00 p.m._____

3:00 p.m._____

4:00 p.m._____

5:00 p.m._____

6:00 p.m._____

7:00 p.m._____

_____

_____

_____

_____

Any format close to this is useful.

2) **Write all entries in *pencil*.** Why? Because things come up in real life, and thus your schedule will need to change. Writing in pencil allows you to erase. Yes, erase—keeping a schedule forces you to see that you cannot "multitask" and do several things at once. Writing one activity in on one space helps to accomplish this. Writing with ink will result in cross-outs and cramming in ever more information.

3) **Keep *one* schedule.** Keep a schedule for *the whole day*, not just your time at work. Activities outside of work should be scheduled, too. This includes picking up children after school or attending an evening meeting at your church or a friend's home. *Keep the schedule with you, on your person.*

4) **Eliminate "to-do lists."** A to-do list is just a list of tasks to be carried out in the future. Why not list *when* you will do each task? That is, put it in your schedule! This will likely help reduce being overly ambitious with your to-do lists and not completing what is intended. Scheduling the task forces you to schedule it when it can be done, which means it will more likely get done. If it is written in pencil, it can easily be rescheduled.

5) **Prioritize.** One problem that contributes to memory problems is scheduling too many daily tasks in addition to routine tasks. Rarely do people complete more than five or six "to-dos" over and above their normal routines. Be realistic with how much time tasks take to do.

6) **Schedule routine events first.** Block off meal times, bed times, and other routine activities to ensure routines can be established. This should be done first. Then, put in special daily events for the upcoming time period (week, month, two months, etc.). Routine events such as meals and bed times should be changed under only extraordinary circumstances.

7) **Schedule the week.** Set aside a regular Saturday or Sunday time to schedule the upcoming week. This does not have to be every activity of every day, just the highlights and important things. Do this at the same time each week (say, Sunday at 5 p.m.) to ensure it will be done and not forgotten.

8) **Use the schedule!** Make a routine where you look at the schedule before or after breakfast or at some starting point of your day. One participant in early MAAT research placed her planner in her bathroom on a shelf each night before she went to bed. In this way, she could not avoid looking at her schedule when she was done with her morning routine. Pair your "schedule looking time" with something you already do at the start of every day.

9) **Simplify.** Keep your schedule simple. Avoid the temptation of scheduling too many tasks. If this happens, look over the schedule in the past week and schedule only those tasks that are most important and that have the greatest likelihood of getting done.

Memory Routines

Memory routines involve always doing things the same way as a regular ritual so that you don't lose things or forget the steps in a task. Examples of memory routines are:

Placing car or house keys on the same hook *every time* you walk in the door
Placing your purse to the right of the chair leg when you sit down
Keeping your day planner or electronic device in the same spot every bedtime (such as the bathroom example we just mentioned)
Having a routine for locking up your office or shop (e.g., shut off computers; check the lights, alarm, door/window locks). The *order is same each day.*

Follow these routines *without exception.*

Object placement areas are sometimes referred to as "memory places" so that you can reliably depend on the locations of objects. Examples include keeping an ID badge in the same spot on your dresser or table when it's not in use and routinely park in the same spot (or close to it).

One tip in starting a new memory place or routine is to place the object or do the task *right before or right after* doing a task you do daily now. For example, to remember the placement of an important object like your car keys, place the keys on the same hook right after walking in the door when getting home, every time. For a new task, such as taking a new daily medicine (such as hormonal therapy after breast cancer), pair taking the medicine with an existing daily task. For example, take the medicine *just before* brushing your teeth. One survivor in past MAAT research attached their toothbrush with Velcro to the medicine bottle. This was also an external cue (discussed in Visit 5) to help establish a new memory routine of taking important medicine. By doing a new task close to something you do routinely every day already, the new task will become habit.

A chart like this can help you establish new memory routines. You need not use this format, but it may be helpful in getting started:

New Object Placement/Routine	Where	When
car keys	*far left hook in mudroom*	*entering house*

Homework

Box 4.1 Memory and Attention Adaptation Strategies, Visit 4

- Keeping a schedule
- Memory routines

The homework to do for the next visit is to implement the daily schedule and try a new memory routine that can simplify your daily life (Box 4.1). As stated earlier, try any routine you think will be most useful to you. Do not feel obligated to try too many at once—one is plenty to start. The point is to do what you feel most comfortable doing and put it into daily life. Once again, you can use the homework task sheet to keep track of the methods you've used. Feel free to read ahead, but don't overwhelm yourself with new information. Simply using this workbook to review what you have learned today is perfectly fine.

Visit 5

In This Visit You Will:

- Review your practice and use of strategies and all skills to date (relaxation, etc.).
- Get introduced to more external strategies (external cueing, distraction reduction, and activity scheduling and pacing) for stress management.
- Apply the new memory and attention strategies in daily life.

Homework Review

The clinician will ask you:

- How does keeping a daily schedule simplify your life? Is your time more manageable?
- Are you looking at the schedule at set times during the day to know what's next? Are you less prone to forget important activities or appointments?
- Are you using a pencil if you have a paper day planner? Is your electronic schedule easiest in day view?
- What memory routine do you now do?
- Is it part of daily life for you?
- Can you use it in another situation?

External Cueing

External cueing is a term psychologists use for visual aids or auditory aids to remind people to do something important—in a sense, "reminders." An example of a visual cue is a sign that reads "Wash your hands before returning to work" or a green or red traffic light. An example of an auditory cue is a beep or tone that reminds you to turn off your headlights, or the ring of a phone.

External cues can help you remember to do important daily tasks such as taking medicine. For example, someone with diabetes could post a sign on the medicine cabinet that reads "1. Finger stick; 2. Blood sugar check; 3. Medication." Someone with memory problems could post a sticky note on the breakfast table that reads "look at your schedule" as a reminder to use their schedule for the day. An auditory cue such as a beeper alert on a watch or other device can be used as a reminder of a brief, scheduled work break. In short, external cues are environmental triggers of desired behavior.

Here are some suggestions for using external cues or "reminders":

1) Get a sense of your daily schedule and situations where paying attention or remembering is a problem.
2) Identify the situation, and see if a note, a sign, or an auditory reminder is best to use. If you use a sign or note, put it where you will read it, such as on the handle of the refrigerator or on a surface where there is nothing else (for instance, the seat of a chair). If you use a tone on your watch, smartphone, or desktop computer, be certain it is loud enough and different enough so it doesn't just blend into the background of other sounds.
3) Simplify. In setting up external cues, use as few words or tones, beeps, etc. as possible. Don't use too many cues; you'll just ignore them. One or two is best.
4) If the cues don't help remind you when to do things, change them! Make them easy, and make sure they are ones you will use. Don't be afraid to change them, especially if they are not helpful.

Distraction Reduction

In this era of electronic communications technology, there are numerous ways in which we can contact others (and they us): mobile phones, voicemail, text messaging, email, videoconferencing, social media, and other communications software. In an instant, you can get answers to questions that suddenly pop into your mind—either from others or from the banks of information available throughout the internet. But a problem arises when someone else's critical and quick need for information is not convenient to you at the moment. Say you're writing an important letter, report, or memo, you've come up with a great idea, and you're putting it into words. Just then, your cellphone interrupts you with an alert, a text message arrives, or an email window pops up, disrupting your train of thought. Then, when you go back to the task at hand, "poof!"—the working memory of that brilliant idea has disappeared.

With what some term the "creeping ivy" of electronics communication into our lives, we have, as a 21st-century culture, made ourselves available, 24/7, to anyone at any time. This is simply not possible. Yet it has become an expectation—purely a false one—of many. This intrusion into our "thinking space" has invaded not only our privacy but also our cognitive abilities. It has robbed us of deep thought and our need to have enough solitude and personal space to complete a thought and work through goal-directed tasks.

The interruptions and distractions discussed here are not trivial in terms of human attention and memory. Dr. Russell Poldrack at the University of California at Los Angeles found that when research participants were asked to complete a single task or a "dual task," they performed about the same—that is, multitasking did not result in much decline in remembering things learned during multitasking. However, brain imaging suggested that, in the dual task situation, research participants appeared to rely more on "habit learning" rather than the deeper declarative memory, or memory that is stored well and can be used in a flexible way in new situations. This is something like learning a new vocabulary word and then using it later with a new meaning: "After the waterfall, the river is *languid* and still" and then, "A *languid* team left the field after a disappointing loss." In short, multitasking and numerous interruptions from electronic devices can lead to "incomplete" learning of new information, making it difficult to recall the information for later use or to apply it in new situations.

The growing numbers of distracted driving laws enacted nationally point to the impact these devices have on divided attention and reduced driving performance. According to data collected by the National Highway Traffic Safety Administration, in 2017 there were 3,166 distracted driving–related deaths of the 34,247 fatalities on U.S. roadways. So, while we have an abundance of information and social connectedness at our fingertips, the risks of electronic device misuse can have a public safety cost as well as causing a decline in some cognitive abilities. An interesting discussion on this topic is by Dr. Calvin Newport of Georgetown University in his book *Deep Work: Rules for Focused Success in a Distracted World*. Dr. Newport outlines how easy it is to get caught up in the distractions of mobile devices and lose the important cognitive skill of sustained attention.

We could discuss at length the negatives of these interruptions and auditory and visual distractions, but it all boils down to using some commonsense approaches to maximize your focus and concentration in learning situations. Here are some practical methods:

- *Auditory distraction.* When doing tasks that require focus, especially driving or operating dangerous tools such as saws or lawnmowers, shut off your cellphone or any other electronic devices that might interrupt you and stow them. Consider keeping the car radio off. If your vehicle has hands-free calling this may reduce the risk of distraction, but talking on the phone is still a distraction from the important task of focusing on the road.

- *Work area auditory distraction.* For those who work in close proximity to others, phone conversations or personal conversations may be a distraction. Try wearing a headset (with white noise, nature sounds, or some other background sound) or musicians' earplugs that reduce sound while still allowing important sounds (for example, your phone, your name) to get through.

- *Social setting auditory distraction.* A complaint among many chemotherapy recipients is they have a difficult time focusing on and understanding conversations with others, especially if other conversations are going on around them—such as in a small group or in a restaurant. Focus on one person at a time, and face them. Use verbal rehearsals to clarify with them what they said, or use the active listening skills discussed later in MAAT.

- *Email.* Email is one of the most abused communication devices we have. Email is not instant messaging; it is just mail. Read it once a day or twice a day at a set time (20 minutes at 8 a.m., say), and then shut it off to keep tones or windows from popping up on your computer screen. If the item someone emails you is that important, they will call. Consider setting an automatic reply on your email account that notifies people that you may not respond promptly due to the amount of email you get. Provide your phone number and instruct the reader to call if the matter is urgent.

- *Mobile phones, texting, pagers, etc.* Unless you are paid to be on call, or your family or friends may need you in an urgent manner (that is, life or death or an important deadline such as a home sale), why not turn these devices off? Texting is a highly efficient and rapid means of communication, but it is a disruption. When engaged in tasks that require your full attention, like driving, keep the device turned off, or respond only when convenient. These interruptions in attention and focus only detract from deeper memory.

- *Visual distractions.* If you get distracted by interesting or new sights, turn your workspace away from windows or doors. Face the wall, or try to arrange a walled-in space if possible. Make sure your workspace is well lit and you can see your work task easily—squinting is a form of muscle tension and can lead to over-arousal, as seen earlier in the discusion on muscle relaxation.

Activity Scheduling and Pacing

Activity scheduling and pacing involves scheduling daily, pleasant activity to improve your mood, attention, and memory. An anxious, irritable, or depressed mood can reduce the brain's ability to focus attention. If attention is not as good as it could be, then information may be lost before it is "stored" in memory. In other words, if we can't pay attention to things, we won't be able to remember them later on.

Many cancer survivors may think, "If I'm not depressed or generally irritable or anxious, why should I bother with pleasant events scheduling?" The answer to this is a little complex but involves prevention. Identifying and doing one or two pleasant activities a day will help control stress, and controlling stress is one way to prevent anxiety, irritability, or depressed mood. As a result, this gives the brain the best chance of performing well with attention and memory. Therefore, we encourage people to schedule daily pleasant events as a way of controlling stress and maintaining or improving mood and attention. Research suggests this method can help cancer survivors improve their attention and memory problems.

Activity scheduling means scheduling any pleasant activity you wish into your daily routine. This fits nicely with keeping your daily schedule and setting realistic goals. We emphasize that activity scheduling also means *activity pacing*. Simply put, pacing means not doing too much, since overwork or excessive demands can lead to stress and then problems with attention and memory. When deciding what pleasant activities to schedule, pick simple tasks that are well within your control—for example, taking an afternoon tea break, listening to a favorite piece of music, going for a walk, exercising, or watching a favorite movie.

You can also schedule small, achievement-oriented chores like cleaning part of the bathroom or ironing a shirt—anything that is small and represents a break in routine. Chores like these may not produce the greatest amount of pleasure, but you can get a sense of achievement or satisfaction in getting a job done.

Finally, other good activities to schedule are quick relaxation breaks or the progressive muscle relaxation exercise.

Here are some suggested steps in activity scheduling. Remember to schedule activity *before* you do it. Don't wait until you are in the mood to do it. Schedule only activities you know you can do with nearly 100% confidence. The reward of a pleasant event only comes *after* the pleasant event. Remember, too, that the weather or other people can change your plans. Therefore, when planning pleasant events, you may want to include backup events in case a friend cannot meet you or the weather turns bad. In this way, you are in control of your activity—not other people or things like the weather.

Activity Scheduling Steps

1) With your schedule, you are likely familiar with your daily routine, wakeup times, mealtimes, working hours, bedtimes. Include weekdays and weekends.

2) Schedule a pleasant activity (as short or as long as desired) each day. Schedule a "backup event" in case things do not go as planned. Keep it simple.

3) Schedule some quick relaxation (as short or as long as desired), perhaps once every hour—this helps with pacing.

4) Keep track of the most pleasant or achievement-oriented events. Write in a simple 0-to-10 rating next to the event in your schedule: 0 = no pleasure or achievement; 10 = most pleasure or achievement imaginable. Remember, not all events are going to be extremes of 0 or 10 in real life; in fact, most of our activity is somewhere in the middle.

Homework

Box 5.1 Memory and Attention Adaptation Strategies, Visit 5

- External cueing
- Distraction reduction
- Activity scheduling and pacing

In today's visit, you learned about using external cues (or sticky notes), how to minimize distractions, and activity scheduling (Box 5.1). Again, don't get overwhelmed. Just use which strategy or parts of strategies you believe are most applicable to your life. Use this workbook as your guide if you forget something. See how the methods work for you, and make modifications as necessary.

Visit 6

In This Visit You Will:

- Review your practice and use of strategies.
- Be introduced to some other strategies: active listening for following social conversation and fatigue management and sleep improvement.
- Practice the new strategies and apply in daily life.

Homework Review

- Does external cuing help you remember to complete important tasks? Is it a strategy that helps your daily life now, or is it something you may use later?

- How about the distraction reduction methods? Are you distracted more by sounds or by visual things? Both? Are you better able to focus and stay on task when you use the distraction reduction methods? What situations require distraction reduction?

- Are you using activity scheduling and pacing? Does scheduling pleasant events help with daily stress? Is pacing sensible for you?

Active Listening

This is similar to verbal rehearsal when meeting individuals and trying to remember their name (as seen in Visit 3). "Active listening" is a term psychologists and other health professionals use when describing interview behaviors. As we discussed earlier, surveys of cancer survivors who have undergone chemotherapy have found that many have difficulty following or understanding conversations when there are several small conversations going on at the same time. In fact, a sizable portion of these survivors report they avoid social activities so they don't look "stupid." Rather than avoid valuable social activities and relationships (such as valued time with friends and loved ones, book clubs, family get-togethers, community and church groups, etc.), using active listening behaviors may help improve involvement and enjoyment. If nothing else, these behaviors can help you clarify and follow conversational content. Here are the basics to try:

1) *Active Listening Behaviors.* Look at the person you are talking to. You don't need to stare or have "fixed-evil-eye" eye contact, but do face them. Keep your

muscles relaxed. Convey body language that lets others know you are engaged with them.

2) *Summarization.* It is alright to summarize what you think you just heard someone say to you—not in vivid detail, but the basic gist. In short, repeat what you just heard. For example, "So you went to the store and found some good bargains."

3) *Clarification.* This is similar to summarization but involves clarifying what you think you heard but weren't sure about. It is OK to clarify by asking a question or prefacing what you want clarified by saying something such as, "Just to be clear," "Did I hear you right?", or simply "I'm sorry, I'm a little confused. Did you say you went to the store on Maple Street and found some good bargains?"

While these active listening skills appear simple, they do take some practice so they go smoothly. The important thing is to try not to avoid situations but to use these skills assertively. All people can have difficulty focusing on conversations, lose their train of thought while speaking, and feel off track. By using these methods in daily conversations, you may be more likely to focus on the things being talked about and store them into memory so that discussion can carry on at a later time.

Fatigue Management and Sleep Improvement

Entire cognitive-behavioral treatments have been developed to improve both fatigue and sleep quality. Sleep difficulty is more common among cancer survivors than the general population, and fatigue remains a problem for many survivors even after treatment is completed. Instead of going into great detail, we will identify the basics of improving sleep quality first, and then we will outline steps to take that may help reduce daytime fatigue. For more detailed information, see the online publication "Facing Forward: Life After Cancer Treatment" at: https://www.cancer.gov/publications/patient-education/facing-forward.

Fatigue Management

Fatigue during chemotherapy is common. For some individuals it can linger for months to a year following the end of treatment, but there is no consistent pattern of fatigue across individuals, and often fatigue improves with time. The exact causes of fatigue associated with cancer treatment are unclear. Some causes may include anemia (reduced red blood cells), nutritional problems, or lack of liquids during cancer treatment, and chronic or persistent pain can make fatigue worse. Also, depression can contribute to fatigue.

Steps for Improved Fatigue Management

1) **Use the pacing methods outlined in the section on activity scheduling.** Breaking up daily tasks into smaller tasks and taking brief breaks will help prevent fatigue from building up. It is important to shift tasks at scheduled times even if you don't feel fatigued. This way, you will likely spread out your valued and busy activity over time and still achieve your goals but with better control of fatigue.

2) **Use relaxation skills.** In particular, be sure to practice quick relaxation through the day—this will help restore energy. Again, don't wait until you are tired or run down; do this at predetermined times.

3) **Take part in sensible exercise.** Many people who have fatigue problems avoid exercise or physical activity thinking it will add to fatigue. In fact, exercise such as walking 30 minutes a day, three or four days per week, can boost energy levels, especially if you pace yourself well. As usual, before beginning any exercise, check with your doctor or health professional. If you are not sure what type of exercise to do, many medical centers have physical therapists or personal trainers in wellness programs who can make good recommendations.

4) **Diet.** Check with a dietitian to see if there are foods you should consume more of to boost energy or if there are foods to avoid that may contribute to fatigue.

5) **Medicines, supplements, or natural substances.** Check with your doctor to see if there are safe medicines that may help with fatigue. Provigil can help with daytime fatigue and may be helpful with cognitive problems. However, medicine may not be for everyone, and there may be other supplements, vitamins, or natural ingredients that can be helpful. As always, alert your health professionals about anything you are taking. Although natural substances are "natural," they are not natural to your body and may interact dangerously with medicines.

Sleep Quality Improvement

Sleep is an important function for optimal health. Adequate sleep quality can boost immune system function and musculoskeletal health and help regulate mood. More pertinent to MAAT, sleep quality can boost and optimize cognitive function—memory and attention. Psychologists, neuroscientists, and other sleep researchers believe that one of the principal functions of sleep is to help the brain get its share of glucose, the sugar-based nutrient that the brain uses for energy. When you're asleep, your body is using much lower levels of glucose, allowing the brain to meet its nutrient needs and restore delicate metabolic balance. With adequate nutrition, the brain has the best chance of maintaining its memory and attention functions.

You are already practicing one method known to enhance sleep quality: progressive muscle relaxation, or the skill of keeping skeletal muscles relaxed. Continue to practice your relaxation skills and apply them to sleep—that is, when you are going to bed, let your muscles relax to the greatest extent possible.

Other steps that research has shown will improve sleep quality are discussed in the following list. The sooner you begin to implement these, the sooner you will see a difference in you sleep quality because these sleep habits will improve sleep over time. It is not as simple as taking a pill. While some medications are certainly helpful for improving sleep quality, many only initiate sleep and don't help sustain it. Further, many medications, when used repeatedly over weeks at a time, can lead to tolerance of the medication, thus requiring more to get its initial effects. Ask your primary care doctor for more information about the benefits or drawbacks of these medications.

Steps for Improved Sleep Quality

1) **The bedroom should be a "dedicated sleep chamber."** Your bedroom or sleep area should be free of wakeful distractions. This is key since the overall goal of these steps is to increase the time spent in bed asleep and not awake. Lying in bed awake only conditions the brain to be awake and promotes excessive worry about not sleeping. Avoid watching television, viewing tablets or mobile phones, or listening to music. Use the bed only for sleeping. Keep it dark when going to bed.

2) **The technology-free sleep chamber.** Blue light emitted by TV, mobile phone, tablet, and computer screens suppresses production of the hormone melatonin, the hormone that helps regulate sleep and wake circadian rhythms. Ideally, these devices should not be in the bedroom. If a mobile device is used as an alarm clock, simply keep the face of the phone downward and ensure all audio alerts are off. Settings or apps on some devices can help promote sleep time. Try not to view devices 45 minutes prior to going to bed. In short, blue light may promote wakefulness in the way daylight might, so a technology-free sleep chamber is a good idea.

3) **Bed times, wake times.** Go to sleep and get up at the same time each day. Having a regular schedule is important to help your brain develop regular sleep stage cycles. However, remember that if you have slept fine for a few days and have trouble sleeping one night, it doesn't necessarily mean your whole cycle will get thrown off. Just continue the schedule as regularly as possible.

4) **Don't lie in bed awake for longer than 25 to 30 minutes.** If this happens, get up and go to another room. Then, do something that is relaxing (read, listen to music, or practice your relaxation skills) and return to bed when you feel sleepy.

5) **Avoid daytime napping.**

6) **Worry time.** If you find yourself habitually thinking about things in bed that produce anxiety, such as what you need to do the next day, start scheduling a few minutes during the day (not before bed) as your "worry time" or time to schedule things you need to do tomorrow. You may conclude you have done all you can that's within your control about the topic of worry, which is a resolution that will allow for the task of sleep.

7) **Wind-down time.** Remember that some people need more time to unwind before bed than others. If you need to, allow yourself an hour (or longer) to unwind before bed—take a bath, read, watch television. Never do work right up until bedtime. Always stop at least 30 minutes to an hour before bed.

8) **Caffeine use.** Avoid caffeinated beverages after 5 p.m.

9) **Exercise schedule: Keep it sensible.** Late-night exercise may be arousing and may make it difficult to fall asleep. However, regular exercise done earlier in the day can help to regulate nighttime sleep.

Homework

Box 6.1 Memory and Attention Adaptation Strategies, Visit 6

- Active listening
- Fatigue management and sleep improvement

In today's visit, you learned about using active listening behaviors to help you re-engage in social activities or focus better in social conversation (Box 6.1). You also learned about how you can use behavioral methods to improve fatigue management and sleep quality. Try one or two of these strategies. Remember, don't become overwhelmed and implement all of them at once. Do what you believe is a priority. Focus on the real-world use and application of the strategy and see how it works. Again, keep track of what you do and review this with your clinician at the next MAAT visit. Feel free to read ahead in the MAAT workbook, but don't overwhelm yourself with too much information.

Visit 7

In This Visit You Will:

- Review your practice and use of active listening and sleep strategies
- Be introduced to visualization strategies (internal strategies)
- Tie in the strategies learned to date
- Practice the new strategies and apply them in daily life

Homework Review

- Are you better able to focus on conversations using active listening strategies? Does active listening help you follow one conversation at a time? More importantly, are you engaging in social activities you value, when you want to? Are you applying decatastrophizing to help you cope with small social mistakes that we all make (such as forgetting a word or name)? Is active listening helping you regain more social activity?

- Are regular bed and wake times helping you to establish a good sleep routine? Are the sleep improvement strategies helping you feel more rested when you wake up? Are you less anxious about sleep?

- Does exercise help with fatigue? Does activity pacing help with fatigue?

Visualization Strategies

Sometimes it is easiest to remember verbal information if you can get a "mental picture" of it. At its simplest, visual imagery uses mental visual pictures that are associated with a person (names), place, or thing or perhaps a task you want to remember. This is nothing new. For years advertisers have found that logos can improve sales of products when a simple visual picture becomes associated with a name. For example, what do you think of when you see golden arches along most North American highways?

Some neuropsychologists believe that by using visual imagery to remember names (places, people, objects), the brain can use circuits in the visual system to aid the auditory-verbal memory system. In a sense, the visual circuitry in the brain may be able to bypass and take over for other regions damaged or affected by cancer and cancer therapy. Some research evidence suggests that using mental pictures can improve word and name recall.

The sections that follow describe a number of visualization methods that can be helpful. You can apply these visualization methods to help you remember passwords and personal identification numbers (PIN). With all the electronic devices we have and the numerous access and security codes we need (PINs for bank accounts, passwords for online accounts, etc.), it is a wonder anyone can keep it all straight! You can also use visual imagery to commit to memory important mobile phone numbers of loved ones, just as you did with the verbal rehearsal strategy. These are just a few of the applications where visual imagery may be helpful.

Here are some methods and how to use them:

Simple Visualization

1) *State the name of what it is you want to remember.* It's always helpful to rehearse something out loud or silently if you want to remember it later. You may even repeat the name, place, or object several times. See if it sounds like something you can picture.

2) *Next, describe what you "picture" or visualize.* When you say the name, place, or object, what do you think of? For example, the word or phrase you want to remember may have a peculiar sound association. For example, the last name Ahles—is a close association to "All-ice." You could picture a person sculpted out of ice. Or a certain place or town may already evoke a visual image—for example, a town called "MacDonald" may evoke visions of a farm or golden arches.

3) *Now exaggerate the image.* Once you think of an image associated with the word or phrase, now make it ridiculous. For example, in the "All-ice" example, you could visualize the person as a giant ice-monster looming over a city. Or picture a giant Statue of Liberty dominating the landscape. If you're trying to remember a PIN, imagine giant numbers of your PIN standing in line at an ATM. The point is that making an image exaggerated, ludicrous, and/or humorous adds to the emotional association—deeper emotion "deepens" the memory. Think of the most embarrassing moment you've ever had, your proudest moment of achievement, or where you were when you heard of the events of September 11, 2001. All have strong emotions associated with them. Therefore, create images that can evoke emotion.

4) *Visualization with a twist.* Finally, you may want to "visualize" smells with names, places, or things. Many people already can instantly identify a flower's name or the name of a spice simply by its smell but not appearance. This is also true of some towns (one author attended public schools in a rural Maine town with a large paper mill that emitted not the most flattering of odors—many people familiar with the town recall the town by its smell, not its beautiful scenery). Use smells to evoke a "mental picture" that fits the word in the same fashion as above.

The Name–Face Mnemonic ("Name–Face Association")

Many of us have trouble from time to time remembering which names go with what face. However, paying attention while looking at a person and attending to hearing their name can help consolidate a memory. An additional strategy, the name–face mnemonic, can also enhance name–face recognition. It has three steps:

1) *Think of a picture that is somehow related to a name.* For example, if you meet someone named "Brooks," you could picture a stream covered with rocks and a grassy bank. If you meet someone called "Winslow," you could associate it with "wind-slow," perhaps picturing a still sailboat adrift with flapping sails.
2) *Examine the person's face for a prominent feature.* Perhaps a nose or a forehead stands out, or their eyes, their hair, or another feature.
3) *Have the prominent feature and the image interact in some way.* Picture the visual image and the prominent feature interacting in some absurd way. For example, you could picture the stream running down Mr. or Ms. Brooks' forehead. The absurd nature of the image evokes more emotion—hopefully humor!—which helps to "deepen" the memory and will enhance the odds of later recall.

As with any verbal memory skill, practice will bring about the best results. Obviously, this strategy is best practiced in public settings where you can meet people. However, there are other ways to practice even if you have few opportunities to socialize and meet new people. Use the name–face mnemonic while watching television news broadcasts (or other programs) and practice remembering the names of the faces you see on screen. You can also practice with photos of people you see online or in magazines if their names are given in captions—anywhere a name–face association can be made. Walk away from the image and keep it pictured in your mind as you repeat the person's name. Come back in five minutes and see if you accurately recalled the name. Now walk away for seven minutes . . . and so on. Be creative in your practice methods.

Method of Loci ("The Journey")

The method of loci or "the journey" (also known as "the mental walk") is another visualization strategy to help you remember lists of words—names of objects, places, people, etc. It may be a useful way to remember a grocery or shopping list, a list of errands or "to-do" items, or new material when taking a class or academic course. It was originally used as a learning skill in ancient Greece, in the days when paper was expensive, so that speakers could remember each point they wanted to make while delivering a speech or lecture. Today, people with superior memory skills who compete in memory competitions use the method of loci.

Using the method of loci is straightforward and similar to the visualization technique we discussed earlier in this chapter.

1) *Picture a familiar space with different rooms.* This is usually done with the first floor of your home or living space, which you have walked through innumerable times. It will serve as a "visual template" in which to "place" the things you want to remember. Picture walking in the entrance you use most often and think of the path you typically follow as you walk through your home (the entryway, the kitchen, a living room to the left, a hall leading to another room, etc.).

2) *In each room, picture one of the objects or items to be remembered.* Here's where your "visual template" comes in handy. For example, we can use a simple grocery list. Picture a large gallon of milk standing in the entryway, a bag of frozen peas sitting on the counter in the kitchen, carrots standing next to the refrigerator, a ball of twine sitting in the living room, and duct tape in the hall.

3) *Once again, make the image of the objects odd or absurd.* Picture a giant gallon of milk with arms and legs and the peas spilled all over the countertop. Again, evoke emotion to "deepen" the memory. Using this type of emotional encoding or "storage method" will deepen the memory and make it easier to recall.

The most important point in using the method of loci is to use the same memory space, such as the rooms of your home, each time you want to remember a list of objects, items, or names. Most people can remember their home well, but it is the list of items or tasks that is new and most easily forgotten. Therefore, you will use the familiar space over and over again but with different objects each time you have a new set of items to remember (such as a shopping list).

If you live in a small apartment with few rooms or an open-plan house, you can use different spaces such as familiar cabinets and drawers, countertops, and closets as the memory space in the method of loci. Another alternative is using a familiar route that you use, such as your commute to work. Some individuals have used their body in the method of loci: They might visualize green beans on their head, tomatoes for a neck, milk balanced on the left shoulder, and so forth. It doesn't matter if your memory space involves rooms, a route, or body parts. The important thing is to keep it simple and to use the same memory space each time you encounter a list of things you want to commit to memory.

A final word on the method of loci: Start by remembering perhaps four rooms or spaces in which to place the objects you wish to remember. Then work up to more spaces as you become familiar with the strategy. Challenge yourself: Try running a few errands without a list. Many people use four or five rooms to remember lists of about that length and then work up to more items. As with anything, practice and daily application will make the strategy simple and easy to use with time, so commit the time to mastering the method.

Homework

Box 7.1 Memory and Attention Adaptation Strategies, Visit 7

- Visualization strategies

In today's visit, you learned about using visualization strategies to pair visual information with other sensory experience (auditory) to improve memory storage and later recall (Box 7.1). Try one or two of these strategies. Once again, keep it simple. Don't become overwhelmed and implement everything at once. Do what you believe works best and is practical for you. Apply these strategies in daily life and see how it works. Again, keep track of what you do and review this with your clinician at the next visit.

Visit 8

In This Visit You Will:

- Review your practice and use of visualization strategies.
- Tie together strategies learned to date.
- Maintain strategies learned and adapt them to future changes.
- Discussion and wrap-up.

Homework Review

- Are you using visualization strategies to help you recall things?

- Are you using them to help you recall names of people you have recently met? How about passwords or personal identification numbers (PINs) for bank accounts, daily tasks or running errands without a list, or any number of similar applications?

- How are you using other strategies at the same time, such as relaxation skills, verbal rehearsal strategies, and using a schedule (day planner)?

Tying Together Strategies and Maintenance

To date, you have learned a number of strategies to help you compensate for and self-manage memory and attention problems related to cancer. These strategies have combined methods that are internal (ones you can use in your mind or with your voice) and external (strategies using devices such as a daily schedule). You have also learned and applied some basic stress management strategies: applied relaxation skills and activity pacing and scheduling. Table 8.1 summarizes all these strategies.

Now that you have learned skills for managing memory and attention problems, the key is to maintain the new behaviors that you have worked hard on acquiring. Research on health behavior change suggests that it takes a number of weeks of daily practice until a new behavior becomes routine. The main points here are:

1) By practicing good memory and attention habits (MAAT strategies), memory and attention failures can be prevented, or, when they do arise, will be better managed.

Table 8.1 MAAT Strategies

Visit 1
  • Self-awareness and monitoring of memory problems
  • Progressive muscle relaxation

Visit 2
  • Quick relaxation
  • Self-Instructional Training

Visit 3
  • Verbal and silent rehearsal
  • Cognitive restructuring or challenging unhelpful thoughts, beliefs, and assumptions

Visit 4
  • Keeping a schedule
  • Memory routines

Visit 5
  • External cueing
  • Distraction reduction
  • Activity scheduling and pacing

Visit 6
  • Active listening
  • Fatigue management and sleep improvement

Visit 7
  • Visualization strategies

2) Memory problems are to be expected, particularly in times of increased stress or when upsetting life events occur. The skills you learned in this program will be most useful when memory difficulties arise.

3) However, an important point is to practice the attention and memory strategies presented in this workbook *on a daily basis.* Do NOT wait until memory and attention problems arise. Once you begin regular use of the skills you learned here to cope with and manage symptoms, dealing with them becomes automatic and natural.

A maintenance plan for maintaining your skills should include the following five points: self-evaluation, the importance of pacing, the importance of practice, review, and the importance of social support.

Point 1: Self-Evaluation

At least once a month, use the Memory and Attention Problem Record for two or three days in a row. You can make additional copies as needed. The reason for this is to look closely at what situations contribute to what types of attention and memory problems. See if the 0-to-10 ratings are lower or higher, and note if stress has an effect on attention and memory. By writing it down, you can take a careful look at what the problem situations are—such as at work or when you are tired—and iden-tify the most effective skills that can help. As life circumstances change (as they do for all of us), we may face different memory demands. Therefore, this self-assessment can be helpful in determining what life changes have taken place and whether they demand different memory skills.

For example, a nurse may have a job that mostly involves administering intra-venous (IV) medications. The nurse may use Self-Instructional Training skills to make sure no steps in the administration process are skipped and no errors are made during IV medication administration. But if the nurse takes a new job that mostly involves conducting educational sessions, such as in a diabetes service, more verbal rehearsal and active listening skills will be important to recall names and teaching points.

Point 2: The Importance of Pacing

If you notice you are increasingly tired or fatigued, you might want to devote more attention to good activity pacing. Activity scheduling and pacing can help with fa-tigue management, as can the relaxation skills you have learned.

Point 3: The Importance of Practice

Using the most valued strategies in this workbook every day is practice. You are encouraged to refine and apply other strategies in addition to the ones (at least two) you are applying every day. However, keep it simple and emphasize the practical.

Point 4: Review

At least once a month, look over this workbook to refresh your understanding of the skills that are most helpful and important to you. Also, look over the other portions of the workbook so that you don't miss information that could be helpful to you. Again, your life circumstances may change with a move, new job, or family circumstances. You thus may have new tasks, routines, or job demands that require different forms of memory. Therefore, strategies that you may not find useful at present may become useful in the future. This monthly review can help you be prepared for such change.

Point 5: The Importance of Social Support

Health psychologists have long known that having regular interaction with loved ones, friends, spouses, neighbors, family, co-workers, or close others can boost many aspects of health. "Social support" has been demonstrated to boost some immune system functions and is associated with longevity. It has also been demonstrated that social support can help people cope with the burden of cancer and maintain new health behaviors. This does not mean you have to have a large network of friends or throngs of admiring community members or fan clubs. You don't have to be the life of the party. Rather, if you are satisfied with the quality of supportive others in your life who have helped you through cancer or other health challenges, or life in general, this would qualify as good social support. To help you maintain the new strategies you have learned with MAAT, talk to your social support network and ask them to help you keep on track. For example, ask them to quiz you to help you remember names or directions and to play games that require memory, vocabulary, and reasoning skills. Take a course together. Try to schedule regular exercise together. You may even share this workbook with your social support network and commit to using strategies together daily, such as use of a daily schedule, activity scheduling, or daily progressive muscle relaxation. In short, social support has many health benefits and often it is cost effective (that is, inexpensive). The key is to reach out and ask—you may also be giving something in return.

Form 8.1 is a written maintenance plan. The point of the form is to have a written plan for maintaining behavioral skills on your own. You should complete this with your clinician. Keep in mind that the point of this plan is to help you keep up with your memory and attention skills always.

The End of the Beginning

As a cognitive-behavioral program, MAAT has covered a lot of material. You have learned about the various effects different forms of cancer and cancer treatments can have on memory and attention and the typical types of memory problems experienced by many individuals who have never had cancer treatments. You have also learned and applied a variety of adaptive strategies to help you improve performance in daily life *where you use your memory*. This is now "the end of the beginning," and now you will begin to refine, reuse, and find creative ways to apply all the MAAT strategies for improving memory function in your daily life.

This visit does not have to be your last contact with the clinician you are seeing. You may, from time to time, if your health or life circumstances change or other factors arise that affect daily memory function, re-consult your clinician for two or three visits for a "booster." This may not be necessary, but in some cases it may be useful. For now, continue with the new strategies and refine their application.

Form 8.1 Maintenance Plan

1. In the table below, list the adaptation strategies you prefer and use most in the left column. In the right column, indicate if you use the strategy daily and under what situations you are likely to use it (for example, work, home, or community). Review this once per month. Revise as needed.

Strategy	When Used, How Often? What Situations?

2. What day and time will you review your MAAT workbook each month?

3. Social support: Who will you use to help you keep on track? When will you use or ask your social support network for help?

Index

Tables and figures are indicated by *t* and *f* following the page number